REVIEW COPY

Please submit two tear sheets of review.

U.S. list price: $52.00

With the compliments of
FUTURA PUBLISHING COMPANY, INC.
135 Bedford Road, PO Box 418,
Armonk, NY 10504-0418
Web Site: www.futuraco.com

A Practical Guide to the Use of the High-Resolution Electrocardiogram

by

Edward J. Berbari, PhD
Professor and Chairman, Electrical Engineering
Professor of Medicine and
Director, Biomedical Engineering
Electrical Engineering Department
Indiana University Purdue University Indianapolis
Indianapolis, Indiana

and

Jonathan S. Steinberg, MD
Chief, Division of Cardiology
Director, Arrhythmia Service
Co-Director, Heart Center
St. Luke's-Roosevelt Hospital Center;
Associate Professor of Medicine
Columbia University College of Physicians and Surgeons
New York City, New York

Futura Publishing Company, Inc.

Library of Congress Cataloging-in-Publication Data

Berbari, Edward J.
    A practical guide to the use of the high-resolution
electrocardiogram / by Edward J. Berbari and Jonathan S.
Steinberg.
        p. cm.
    Includes bibliographical references and index.
    ISBN 0-87993-445-X (alk. paper)
        1. Electrocardiography.   2. Electrocardiography—Data
processing.   I. Steinberg, Jonathan S.   II. Title.
        [DNLM: 1. Electrocardiography—methods.   WG 140 B484p
2000]
    RC683.5.E5 B418 2000
    616.1′207547—dc21
    DNLM/DLC
    for Library of Congress   99–052567
                                                                            CIP

Copyright © 2000
Futura Publishing Company, Inc.

Published by
Futura Publishing Company
135 Bedford Road
Armonk, New York 10504

LC#: 99-052567
ISBN#: 0-87993-445-X

*My wife, Terry, and four children
(Nicolas, Jonathon, Kathleen, and
Michael) have tolerated my Sunday
evening work schedule for many years.
Without this support and understanding,
this special time would not be available.
It has enabled me to write this book and
I am sincerely thankful for their sacrifice.*
—EJB

---

*To my wife and best friend, Alice, and
my children (my other best friends),
Rachel and Joshua, for giving me the
support and encouragement to make this
work possible.*
—JSS

Preface

The specialty of cardiac electrophysiology is advancing at a rapid and unprecedented pace. Astounding progress has been made over the past three decades, resulting in a better understanding of the genesis of a variety of arrhythmias and the underlying electrophysiological-anatomic substrate for these arrhythmias, use of appropriate models to predict which patients are at greater risk, and a vast array of treatment modalities.

Although many aspects of clinical electrophysiology take place in the invasive laboratory, noninvasive techniques continue to play a fundamental and important role. Of course, the most basic electrophysiological technique is the electrocardiogram. Computer enhancement of the electrocardiogram to permit body surface recording of small-amplitude cardiac signals was a major advance. This technique, known as the high-resolution (or signal-averaged) electrocardiogram, greatly facilitated the collection of critical electrophysiological data heretofore obtainable only by invasive techniques. Based on exhaustive and comprehensive clinical studies, from a foundation of experimental work, the high-resolution electrocardiogram can play a critical role in the identification of clinical subsets at high risk for ventricular arrhythmias and for a better understanding of these arrhythmias.

The purpose of this book is to provide an up-to-date and comprehensive review of high-resolution electrocardiography. The subject matter, however, has been selected to highlight the background and application of aspects of high-resolution electrocardiography that have a practical use. Initial chapters deal with the background and the underlying pathophysiology of cardiac late potentials. The middle chapters deal with the technical aspects of acquisition and analysis of the SAECG. The chapter that follows reviews currently accepted clinical uses for the high-resolution electrocardiogram. Finally, the book concludes with segments on evolving and future uses of these specialized techniques and case studies. Necessarily, a focus of much of the book is on the signal-averaged electrocardiogram and its use for detection of prolonged ventricular activation and the ventricular late potential.

v

This book was made possible through the collaboration of a clinician and a research scientist, both of whom have dedicated substantial parts of their careers to furthering an understanding of arrhythmogenesis, and the ability to pursue this objective through noninvasive techniques. The authors fully expect that this field will continue to move forward with improved utilization of existing techniques and the development of new applications for different patient populations.

Jonathan S. Steinberg, MD

Edward J. Berbari, PhD

Contents

Preface v

1 Introduction 1

2 Pathophysiological Basis of Conduction Delay Detected
   on the Signal-Averaged Electrocardiogram 7

3 Methods for Recording Late Potentials on the
   Body Surface 21

4 Analyzing the Signal-Averaged Electrocardiogram 41

5 The Normal Signal-Averaged Electrocardiogram,
   Technical Problems, Pitfalls, and Limitations 63

6 The Signal-Averaged Electrocardiogram in Clinical
   Practice 83

7 Case Studies 147

8 Future Applications of the High-Resolution
   Electrocardiogram 163

   Index 177

1

Introduction

The high-resolution electrocardiogram (ECG) is defined as a body surface electrocardiographic recording that registers cardiac events not seen in the standard ECG. This is usually done by increasing both the time and the voltage scales of the recording instrumentation. These are relatively simple procedures because the ECG is not a technologically difficult signal to record. However, as the ECG signal is amplified, there are sources of noise that can obscure very small cardiac signals. There are several possible sources of interfering noise, but the most significant of these noise signals are the electromyographic (EMG) signals from the skeletal muscles.

Computer-based methods, which will be discussed in later chapters, can be used to decrease the effects of interfering noise signals. The most common method is known as signal averaging. Hence, the term signal-averaged ECG or SAECG is often used interchangeably with the term high-resolution ECG. However, the SAECG is only one method (albeit the primary method used in clinical practice today) for recording a high-resolution ECG.

Briefly, signal averaging requires that the signal of interest be repeated (like the ECG) and that the interfering noise be random. Using computer methods, each QRS can be identified, aligned, and averaged on a point-by-point basis. This reduces the noise and preserves the signal of interest, thus allowing identification of minuscule signals. For example, the typical QRS amplitude is 1.0 mV, and with signal averaging one can identify signals as small as 1.0 μV: 1/1000 of the typical QRS.

Signal averaging was first used to enhance the detection of radar signals and found its first medical application to record electroencephalographic (EEG) signals in the early 1950s. This approach for recording elicited EEG signals from the sensory cortex was first performed on a computer of averaged transients or CAT scope.[1] Some of the low-level EEG signals could be enhanced with signal averag-

1

ing, and the whole field of sensory evoked potentials arose in the 1950s and continues today in the field of diagnostic neurology. The first application of signal averaging to the ECG was perhaps the study of Hon and Lee[2] who were recording the fetal ECG, where the maternal ECG was considered an interfering signal, as well as the fact that it was a relatively smaller signal. Other early ECG applications of signal averaging were reported,[3,4] but the primary interest was the enhancement of the standard ECG waves, e.g., P wave enhancement.

In 1973, Berbari et al.[5] first reported the use of the SAECG to noninvasively record signals from the His-Purkinje system. Numerous other studies followed that also demonstrated the ability to record signals of such a small magnitude. This new methodology, requiring computer processing, had numerous other applications. The noninvasive recording of His-Purkinje potentials has some problems and therefore has not been a common application of the SAECG. Chief among them is the apparent overlap of the terminal portion of the P wave and beginning of the His-Purkinje waveform in the high-resolution mode. These limitations were observed during the early development of the SAECG and newer approaches in signal processing may warrant a reexamination of this application. However, its clinical usefulness needs to be firmly established.

This initial application of the SAECG came a few years after the development of invasive cardiac electrophysiology during the era of His bundle electrocardiography. It was hoped that the noninvasive evaluation of the cardiac conduction system would obviate the need for invasive evaluation. However, both approaches had as their primary clinical goal the identification of patients with intermittent heart block who would have a need for a cardiac pacemaker. Neither method was eventually used for this purpose, and both approaches, the SAECG and invasive cardiac electrophysiology studies, evolved into far more advanced clinical problems.

In the early 1970s, several investigators, studying arrhythmogenic mechanisms in canine infarct models, found that there were measurable and repeatable epicardial signals that extended well beyond the QRS complex.[6,7] In some cases, these potentials extended throughout the diastolic interval exhibiting continuous electrical activity coupling a premature ventricular with the preceding sinus beat.[8] These so-called "late potentials" were measurable on the heart surface, but were not evident in the surface ECG. During the 1970s and 1980s, clinical electrophysiology expanded very rapidly and a primary interest was the identification and therapeutic approach to ventricular tachycardia via programmed ventricular stimulation. Numerous catheters were placed within the ventricles and it was shown that indeed these late potentials were present in humans.

Working in the laboratories of Drs. Benjamin J. Scherlag and Ralph Lazzara, where several of the initial late potential studies were performed, Dr. Berbari extended the SAECG to record the late potentials noninvasively.[9] This initial study in a canine infarct model was followed by a report demonstrating that body surface late potentials could be recorded in humans.[10] A landmark report by Simson[11] in 1981 formalized an approach for recording late potentials and, more importantly, demonstrated their clinical importance by correlating their presence with the inducibility of ventricular tachycardia. Many aspects of the approaches used today for recording cardiac late potentials stem from the early, initial clinical study by Simson.

There were a number of early reports on late potentials, but they suffered from a lack of uniformity in their technology, making comparisons among them difficult. There are now hundreds of papers in the literature covering a wide spectrum of topics using the SAECG to record cardiac late potentials. As a tool, the SAECG has been applied to a number of disease entities. Its primary use has been the identification of patients who have had a prior myocardial infarction, and are at increased risk of life-threatening ventricular tachycardia and sudden death.

There have been a several reviews of the SAECG in the literature. These include the books edited by El-Sherif and Turitto[12] and Gomes.[13] Both are advanced, research oriented reviews. In addition, there was a combined American Heart Association, American College of Cardiology, and European Society of Cardiology Task Force Report that was published in each group's respective journal.[14] A more recent report by an expert committee of the American College of Cardiology also provides guidelines for clinical use.[15] A Technical Information Report from the American Association for the Advancement of Medical Instrumentation[16] was published in 1998 that specifies the technical characteristics of SAECG systems.

Cardiac sudden death claims as many lives each year in the United States as all forms of cancer. Most of these sudden deaths are considered to be arrhythmogenic. The role of the SAECG in identifying patients at risk seems to be an expanding one. Briefly, a positive SAECG recording for cardiac late potentials determines the presence of an arrhythmic substrate. This substrate is most likely the presence of viable but abnormal cells within and around the scarred region of a myocardial infarction. The mere presence of the substrate seems to be a significant risk factor for identifying patients prone to ventricular tachycardia and sudden cardiac death.

There are numerous noninvasive risk factors for sudden cardiac death. Nonalterable ones are family history, age, and gender. Others are disease related, e.g., coronary artery disease, hypertension, and diabetes. Still others are lifestyle dependent, e.g., smoking, cholesterol, and obesity, and these factors can be altered. Another group of risk factors is based on diagnostic tests that usually aim to identify some mechanism underlying the cause of sudden death. Included in this group are cardiac output or other measures of ventricular performance, ventricular ectopy as measured on the ambulatory ECG, cardiac late potentials measured with the SAECG, or inducibility of ventricular tachycardia observed during an electrophysiological study. Hence, the role of the SAECG and its measurement of cardiac late potentials fits in as one piece of the risk stratification puzzle. As we develop the pathophysiological basis of late potentials and examine the large clinical database using late potentials, we will gain a fuller appreciation of the use of this powerful, inexpensive, and noninvasive tool.

References

1. Brazier MAB. Evoked responses recorded from the depths of the human brain. Ann NY Acad Sci 112:33, 1964.
2. Hon EH, Lee ST. Noise reduction in fetal electrocardiography. Am J Obstet Gynecol 87:1086, 1963.
3. Pryor TA, Ridges JG. A computer program for stress test data processing. Comput Biomed Res 7:360, 1974.
4. Brody DA, Woolsey MD, Arzbaecher RC. Application of computer techniques to the detection and analysis of spontaneous P wave variation. Circulation 36:359, 1974.
5. Berbari EJ, Lazzara R, Samet P, Scherlag BJ. Noninvasive technique for detection of electrical activity during the P-R segment. Circulation 48:1005-1013, 1973.
6. Waldo AL, Kaiser GA. A study of ventricular arrhythmias associated with acute myocardial infarction in the canine heart. Circulation 47:1220-1228, 1973.
7. Boineau JP, Cox JL. A slow ventricular activation in acute myocardial infarction: A source of reentrant ventricular contractions. Circulation 48:702-713, 1973.
8. Scherlag BJ, El-Sherif N, Hope RR, Lazzara R. Characterization and localization of ventricular arrhythmias due to myocardial ischemia and infarction. Circ Res 35:372-383, 1974.
9. Berbari EJ, Scherlag BJ, Hope RR, Lazzara R. Recordings from the body surface of arrhythmogenic ventricular activity during the S-T segment. Am J Cardiol 41:697-702, 1978.

10. Rozanski JJ, Mortara D, Myerburg RJ, Castellanos A. Body surface detection of delayed depolarizations in patients with recurrent ventricular tachycardia and left ventricular aneurysm. Circulation 63:1172-1178, 1981.
11. Simson MB. Use of signals in the terminal QRS complex to identify patients with ventricular tachycardia after myocardial infarction. Circulation 64:235, 1981.
12. El-Sherif N, Turrito G (eds). High Resolution Electrocardiography, Futura Publishing Co., Mt. Kisco, NY, 1992.
13. Gomes JA (ed). Signal Averaged Electrocardiography, Kluwer Academic Publ, Dordrecht, Germany, 1993.
14. Breithardt G, Cain ME, El-Sherif N, Flowers N, Hombach V, Janse M, Simson MB, Steinbeck G. Standards for analysis of ventricular late potentials using high resolution or signal-averaged electrocardiography: A statement by a Task Force Committee between the European Society of Cardiology, the American Heart Association, and the American College of Cardiology. Eur Heart J 12:473-480, 1991; Circulation 83:1481-1488, 1991; and J Am Coll Cardiol 17:999-1006, 1991.
15. Cain ME, Anderson JL, Arnsdorf MF, et al. American College of Cardiology expert consensus document: Signal-averaged electrocardiography. J Am Coll Cardiol 27:238-249, 1996.
16. Technical Information Report of the Signal-Averaged ECG Subcommittee of the American Association for the Advancement of Medical Instrumentation (AAMI). TIR, 1998.

2

Pathophysiological Basis of Conduction Delay Detected on the Signal-Averaged Electrocardiogram

Reentry as the Basis for Sustained Ventricular Tachycardia after Myocardial Infarction

The mechanism of sustained ventricular tachyarrhythmias after the acute phase of myocardial infarction has been of intense interest for many years. These arrhythmias may account for cardiac deaths, and a thorough understanding of their mechanisms would likely have important clinical implications for treatment and prevention. Investigation has been accomplished via several different animal models that have provided extensive details of the process of arrhythmia formation and provided a basis for pursuit of these same goals in the more challenging clinical realm.

The possible mechanisms for sustained ventricular arrhythmias are several and include abnormal automaticity, triggered arrhythmias, as well as reentry. The bulk of the evidence strongly supports the notion that reentry is responsible for the majority of arrhythmias that occur after healed myocardial infarction. Reentry requires several electrophysiological conditions to exist so that a circuit can form and be perpetuated as a sustained arrhythmia. These conditions include unidirectional block, slow conduction through at least part of the circuit, and arrival of the wavefront to tissue that has recovered excitability. The presence of slow conduction is a crucial component of the reentrant process.

Complete mapping of the reentrant circuit is difficult under any circumstances, even in experimental models, often because of the

7

small size and ill-defined and unpredictable course of the reentrant circuit. Evidence supporting reentry exists in several forms. The initiation of the tachycardia often develops with premature beats (either spontaneous or artificial), which enhances conduction delay. Laboratory observations have demonstrated greater and greater degrees of conduction delay preceding the ultimate expression of the reentrant tachycardia. At the onset of the tachycardia, continuous electrical activity has sometimes been observed and is thought to represent recording of the entire activation process through the components of the local reentrant circuit. During sustained tachycardias, stimulation with pacing trains or premature beats can reset or entrain the tachycardia, providing additional support for the hypothesis that reentry is present.

Abnormal Ventricular Activation During Normal Sinus Rhythm

It is abundantly clear from multiple sources that the normal myocardial activation process is modified and permanently disrupted by myocardial infarction. Using time domain techniques, the SAECG simply measures prolongation of ventricular activation, and if a late potential is present, it suggests that there are areas of myocardium that are being activated late in the depolarization process relative to the greater bulk of ventricular myocardium. What is the process responsible for this delayed activation and how does it contribute to the risk of reentrant ventricular arrhythmias?

When myocardial infarction occurs, healing is associated with replacement of necrotic tissue with fibrous scar tissue. If the scar tissue is homogeneous and no living myocardial fibers are present, no electrical activity can be recorded from this region. In a transmural myocardial infarction, the central infarct area may exist as such. But many myocardial infarctions are nontransmural, and in addition, all myocardial infarctions have at least some nontransmural areas located in the border regions. In these areas, viable and functional myocardial fibers coexist with fibrous scar tissue. Scar tissue often interdigitates between muscle fibers disrupting the normal parallel pattern of myocardial fiber arrangement as shown in Figure 2.1. In doing so, the fibrous tissue separates myocardial fibers and disrupts the normal intercellular connections that previously existed. Impulses conducting through these regions may be slowed or delayed on the basis of this pathoanatomy. Delayed activation, however, is not synonymous with slow conduction. Individual myocardial fibers,

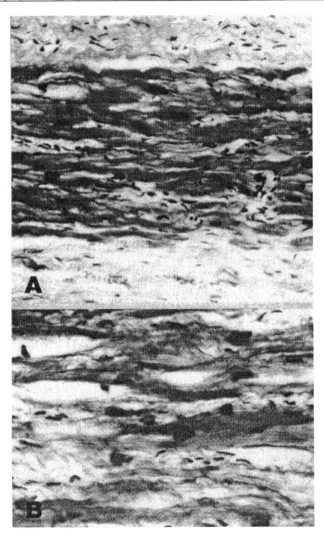

Figure 2.1. The top panel shows tightly packed bundles of myocardial cells. The bottom panel reveals separation of myocardial cells by interstitial connective tissue. (Reprinted with permission from Fenoglio et al. Circulation 68:518.)

when studied from this region, will exhibit normal electrophysiological properties, specifically normal upstroke of the action potential, the depolarization phase. However, conduction may be slowed through this region due to diminished conduction velocity, probably on the basis of anisotropic conduction, which is the slowing of conduction when impulses are forced to propagate transversely across myocardial fibers because of a loss of the normal parallel arrangement. The absence of dense intercellular connections that are normally present between myocardial fibers will directly slow conduction as well. Activation may thus be delayed because of slow conduction. Alternatively, delayed activation of specific components of ventricular myocardial tissue may occur because impulses are forced to propagate through altered pathways that are lengthened by the scarring process.

In healed myocardial infarction, fractionated electrograms are commonly recorded from multiple areas that border on infarcted tissue. These can be recorded through a variety of techniques both experimentally and clinically. Fractionated electrograms are commonly defined as low-amplitude, prolonged, and fragmented local recordings. These electrograms do not per se represent slow myocardial conduction. However, fractionated electrograms probably occur on the same electrophysiological basis as slow conduction and delayed activation in ventricular myocardium.[1] Growth of fibrous tissue leading to separation of myocardial fibers leads to local asynchronous activation of the surviving myocardial fibers that will be represented on a local electrode as a fractionated electrogram. An important concept to keep in mind is that the processes underlying the development of abnormalities in local conduction are the same that would predispose to reentrant ventricular arrhythmias. In fact, more profound and more diffuse abnormal electrograms are found in patients with sustained ventricular tachycardia than in those who have not experienced sustained ventricular tachycardia.[2] These local recordings may be a nonspecific indication that fixed conditions exist for reentry to occur. The more sites that possess these conditions, as well as the presence of the necessary triggers, or modifying factors, the greater the likelihood for ventricular tachycardia.

Relationship of Myocardial Conduction Delay to the Late Potential Recorded with Signal-Averaged Electrocardiograms

Signal-averaged techniques to record late cardiac electrical activity were first performed by Berbari et al.[3] in the first series of canine experiments. These experiments indicated that in the absence of myocardial infarction, signal-averaging did not show any late potential activity on a single surface ECG lead. After experimental infarction, some of the preparations clearly exhibited late potential activity that correlated in time with epicardial activity recorded directly from the heart. Perturbations of the late activity by pacing and by premature beats produced parallel changes on the body surface and on the epicardial surface. With the development of presumed ventricular premature beats, the epicardial electrograms exhibited late potentials. On the SAECG, similar activity at the termination of the QRS (Figure 2.2) was observed. These signals, in the microvolt range and visible only after signal averaging, emphasized the critical need for noise reduction to detect low-amplitude signals not recording directly from the cardiac surface. Also emphasized was the need for high-pass filtering to eliminate the large amplitude ST segment that can become particularly prominent after myocardial infarction; this repolarization phenomenon may mask the presence of low-amplitude depolarization activity when the timing is closely related.

In the controlled conditions of the experimental laboratory, it has also been shown that the SAECG can also reliably establish the

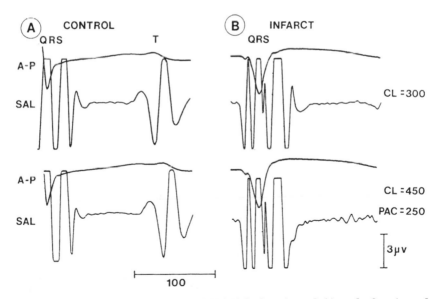

Figure 2.2. Signal-averaged lead (SAL) before (panel **A**) and after (panel **B**) experimental myocardial infarction. Top waveforms were recorded during constant pacing (CL=300 msec) and bottom waveforms following premature atrial complex (PAL). Note multiphasic low-amplitude activity simultaneous with ST segment. (Reprinted with permission from Berbari et al. Am J Cardiol 41:697.[3])

extent of delayed electrical activity that is created by the infarction process.[4] SAECG recordings are sensitive enough to pick up microvolt-level signals even when they occur just after the offset of the QRS. Experimentally, the SAECG has a high sensitivity for detecting any late epicardial activity that can be recorded. In one study,[4] the duration of the signal-averaged lead was closely correlated to the total duration of electrographic activity recorded from infarcted myocardium as shown in Figure 2.3.

The presence of delayed potentials on the SAECG and their relationship to fragmented delayed electrograms suggested the possibility of predicting reentrant ventricular tachyarrhythmias. Several studies using a variety of experimental animal preparations have confirmed this hypothesis. The foundation for use of the SAECG to predict the presence of sustained ventricular tachycardia was established in these experiments. Findings in several studies[5-8] have consistently demonstrated that greater degrees of abnormality on the surface as detected by signal averaging were associated with induction of ven-

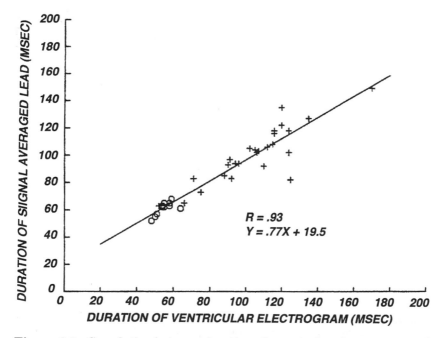

Figure 2.3. Correlation between duration of ventricular electrograms and duration of filtered signal-averaged leads, including controls (open circles) and observations after experimental myocardial infarction (+). (Reprinted with permission from Simson et al. Am J Physiol 1981:H363.)

tricular tachycardia by electrophysiological techniques. The absence of inducible ventricular tachycardia was generally associated with shorter total QRS durations on the SAECG and a lower frequency of late potential or a higher measured voltage in the terminal segment of the QRS. These observations are of course reminiscent of those that have been well demonstrated in the clinical arena.

These experiments have also taught clinicians that it is not reliably possible to accentuate the presence of late potentials by pacing at higher rates or with supraventricular premature beats[5] because there is a variable change in conduction or minimal change in conduction that cannot be detected on the body surface.

In an unstable period during the healing process after experimental infarction, the presence of inducible ventricular tachycardia shows day-to-day variability. The presence of ventricular tachycardia closely correlates with the presence of conduction delay and can be tracked by the SAECG.[6,8] The SAECG thus appears to be a sensitive measure of at least one requirement for the development of ventricular reentry. Experimental infarction models, as well as human myocardial infarction, demonstrated a time-dependent decrease in clinical and inducible ventricular tachycardia. Clearly, the evolution of the pathology of infarct involves changes in ventricular conduction as indicated by the SAECG.

It is clear that myocardial infarction does prolong the signal-averaged QRS duration.[7,8] The degree of QRS prolongation is also related to the extent of myocardial infarction: the larger the myocardial infarction, the longer the filtered QRS duration.[8] In fact, small infarctions or prolonged ischemia alone without sizable infarction do not progress to abnormal SAECG results.[8] In these same animal models, it is more likely to induce sustained ventricular tachycardia in the setting of a large myocardial infarction as measured by various infarct sizing techniques. Among those with large infarctions, the SAECG is able to discriminate which animals will have sustained ventricular tachycardia.[8] SAECG can detect electrophysiological substrate required for reentrant ventricular tachycardia in these animal models with excellent sensitivity and specificity.[7,8]

The previous sections highlight the fact that most ventricular arrhythmias occur on the basis of reentry, that abnormal ventricular activation is frequently found in patients with ventricular tachycardia, and that abnormal ventricular activation is a likely critical component in the development of reentrant ventricular arrhythmias. As will be learned in later chapters, the SAECG is also typically abnormal in patients after myocardial infarction who have ventricular tachycardia. Do the late potentials recorded on SAECG correlate with the abnormal ventricular activation patterns recorded locally?

Necrosis of myocardial tissue and replacement with fibrous tissue leads to a reduction in the amplitude of locally recorded electrograms. Less myocardial tissue undergoes activation per unit time because of the circuitous path the impulse travels or the smaller volume of tissue still viable. The inherent low amplitude of these recordings make enhancement and high resolution a necessity for their accurate representation on the body surface.

What cardiac activity actually gives rise to the late potential on the body surface SAECG? In carefully performed mapping experiments of canine models of reentry in which surviving epicardial tissue forms the substrate for arrhythmia formation, it has been shown that late potentials correlate in time with late-activated epicardial segments.[9] However, not all of the epicardial wavefront was registered on the surface SAECG. The interval after the late potential that gave the impression of electrical quiescence (in reference to depolarization) corresponded to slow conduction and to low amplitude (<0.1 mV) electrograms.[9] The epicardial signals did not exceed the threshold for visualization and detection imposed by background noise in the surface high-resolution ECG.

These observations emphasize the need for optimal noise reduction but also point out that cardiac signals may be so small (<1 mV RMS) that they go undetected on the body surface. These possibilities are in accord with the previous anatomic description of the site of origin of ventricular tachycardia where muscle fibers are separated by fibrous tissue and are located in the border zone of the myocardial infarction.[10] Thus, late potentials correlate in time with delayed ventricular activation, and signal averaging for noise reduction is needed to maximize detection because the late activated sites have a small mass relative to total ventricular mass and give rise to small signals relative to the QRS.

Simson et al.[1] examined direct endocardial and epicardial recordings in patients undergoing cardiac surgery and correlated these recordings with the SAECG. Fragmented electrograms were recorded within areas of previous infarction in patients with and without ventricular tachycardia. However, those with ventricular tachycardia had more sites with fragmented electrograms, and the overall duration of these electrograms was significantly longer. During the main deflection of the QRS, i.e., during its early segment, many electrograms were recorded; these exhibited normal duration, amplitude, and frequency characteristics. When fragmented electrograms occurred during this period, they tended to be short-lived. At the end of the QRS, during the late potential, very few normal electrograms were recorded and instead, activation at this time was dominated by prolonged and fragmented electrograms. Late fragmented electrograms outlasted the normal electrograms by more than 50 msec in the patients who exhibited late potentials. The QRS amplitude on the SAECG correlated with the number of recording sites that demonstrated active electrograms at a particular point in time; the low-amplitude late potential was associated with low-amplitude fractionated electrograms and accurately reflected the volume of abnormal endocardial activity. When patients had no late potentials, there were fewer fragmented electrograms, and most importantly, they were buried within a larger volume of normal electrograms occurring during the earlier segments of the QRS. The terminal portion of the SAECG was more likely to be abnormal when more intracardiac electrograms were recorded late in the sequence of activation, when the termination of these electrograms were delayed, and when these electrograms were abnormal and fractionated.[11]

Simson's work indicated that slow ventricular conduction must result in delayed activation that outlasted normal ventricular depolarization to be identified on the SAECG.[1] Abnormal electrograms that were brief or occurred within the main deflection(s) of the QRS cannot be detected on the SAECG. When they are prolonged and exist at multiple sites, and when they outlast the normal QRS, they can appear on the body surface. Nonetheless, the sites have low amplitude, individually and in aggregate, and thus result in a low-amplitude signal on the body surface. Importantly, it was the abnormal signals that correlated in time with the late potentials on the SAECG, strongly suggesting that they in fact were responsible for the late potential recording.

In a similar study,[12] patients with ventricular tachycardia who underwent endocardial mapping had detailed analyses of endocardial border zone electrograms, which were correlated with the results of SAECG recording. The presence of late potentials was related to the number of sites that exhibited prolonged duration of local electrograms of at least 30 msec. A strong relationship was observed between the number of prolonged electrograms that extended beyond the end of the standard QRS and late potentials; patients with late potentials had more than six times as many sites exhibiting late endocardial electrograms. Similar results have been described during endocardial catheter mapping:[13] patients with signal-averaged late potentials had a greater number of late activated sites that lasted longer relative to the end of the surface QRS. Therefore, it seems likely that a minimal volume of myocardial tissue must undergo late activation in order for the signal to be of sufficient magnitude to be registered, even with signal averaging, on the body surface.

The duration and amplitude of the late potential on the SAECG correlates poorly with similar quantified measures from endocardial recordings.[12] A large number of technical constraints likely contribute to this poor correlation, but do not detract from the important relationship between the presence of a signal-averaged late potential and abnormal endocardial recording. All studies such as these suffer a common limitation in that they clearly represent investigation of a highly select group of patients referred for surgery of ventricular tachycardia. In contrast to animal studies, the number of recording sites was greatly limited and thus minimized the conduction characteristics that were measured and sampled accurately.

Loss of late potentials after interventions that specifically interrupt the process of delayed activation would provide insight into the origins of late potentials. Rozanski et al.[14] were the first to demonstrate quite convincingly that surgical excision by aneurysmectomy and ventriculotomy resulted in complete loss of previously recorded late potentials. Presumably, the critical mass of late activated tissue that had been previously responsible for the late potential had been removed surgically. Whether late activating myocardial tissue was still present but of insufficient magnitude to produce a surface ECG late potential was unknown. But these patients did not have ventricular tachycardia postoperatively, suggesting that the tissue responsible for the late potential, as well as for ventricular tachycardia, had both (or simultaneously) been successfully removed. Interestingly, it is only the surgical removal of wide areas of tissue that abolishes late potentials.[15] Administration of intracoronary ethanol or radiofrequency energy as part of catheter ablation procedures do not consistently eliminate late potentials despite successful outcomes of the procedure.[16,17]

The relationship of SAECG results with the outcome of surgical ablation has important implications. The absence of late potentials after surgery predicts a negative electrophysiological study and thus a benign prognosis.[15,18] The persistence of late potentials is associated with an increased likelihood of the persistence of ventricular tachycardia inducibility and thus the recurrence of ventricular tachycardia. These findings strongly imply that late potentials reflect arrhythmogenic substrate, not simply late endocardial activity, but more detailed mapping may be required to understand this relationship more fully.

Does myocardial tissue that generates the late potential on the SAECG participate in or, in fact, cause the reentrant circuit? This is a difficult question to pursue in clinical models. It is problematic to completely map reentrant circuits with an electrode density sufficient to generate detailed activation maps. A recent analysis[19] shed some light on these issues. Patients undergoing surgery for ventricular tachycardia had detailed three-dimensional activation maps analyzed during sinus rhythm and during ventricular tachycardia; activation times were correlated with SAECG tracings to determine whether the late potential was in fact registered on the basis of activation of myocardial tissue that ultimately participated in ventricular tachycardia. The study found that the vast majority of tissue responsible for a variety of ventricular tachycardias fell within the early and middle portions of the QRS and in only rare instances extended into the terminal portion of the QRS. Furthermore, sites that generated signals during the late portion of the QRS and ST segment were caused by activation of epicardial sites that were in fact related to infarction areas, but were not related to ventricular tachycardia. Unfortunately, the study was greatly limited by the fact that only three patients did not have a bundle branch block and only one of the three had a late potential. Extrapolating these observations to the broader population of patients with ventricular tachycardia would be difficult without larger studies. Nonetheless, similar inferences were drawn from animal work performed by El-Sherif et al.[9] and catheter mapping results in patients with ventricular tachycardia.[13]

The importance of more refined analyses of the SAECG is clear. Reliance on the terminal segment of the signal-averaged QRS leads to definite and predictable limitations. Although use of a total duration overcomes some of these inherent problems, a more thorough look "into the QRS" would be useful. One can safely conclude that the SAECG is a reasonable measure of the overall conduction delay present during myocardial activation. One cannot expect to specifically identify, with 100% accuracy, the probability that this conduction delay will cause reentry or reflect the reentrant myocardial tissue.

References

1. Simson MB, Untereker WJ, Spielman SR, Horowitz LN, Marcus NH, Falcone RA, Harken AH, Josephson ME. Relation between late poten-

tials on the body surface and directly recorded fragmented electrograms in patients with ventricular tachycardia. Am J Cardiol 51:105-112, 1983.

2. Klein H, Karp RB, Kouchoukos NT, Zorn GL, James TN, Waldo AL. Intraoperative electrophysiologic mapping of the ventricles during sinus rhythm in patients with a previous myocardial infarction. Circulation 66:847-853, 1982.

3. Berbari EJ, Scherlag J, Hope RR, Lazzara R. Recording from the body surface of arrhythmogenic ventricular activity during the S-T segment. Am J Cardiol 41:697-702, 1978.

4. Simson MB, Euler D, Michelson EL, Falcone RA, Spear JF, Moore EN. Detection of delayed ventricular activation on the body surface in dogs. Am J Physiol H363-H369, 1981.

5. Spear JF, Richards DA, Blake GJ, Simson MB, Moore EN. The effects of premature stimulation of the His bundle on epicardial activation and body surface late potentials in dogs susceptible to sustained ventricular tachyarrhythmias. Circulation 72:214-224, 1985.

6. Kuchar DL, Rosenbaum DS, Ruskin J, Garan H. Late potentials on the signal-averaged electrocardiogram after canine myocardial infarction: Correlation with induced ventricular arrhythmias during the healing phase. J Am Coll Cardiol 15:1365-1373, 1990.

7. Yoh S, Agawa S, Satoh Y, Furuno I, Saeki K, Sadanaga T, Nakamura Y. Electrophysiological and anatomical substrates for late potential recorded by signal averaging in seven-day-old myocardial infarction in dogs. PACE 13:469-479, 1990.

8. Steinberg JS, Smith R, Bigger JT, Jr, Damm CJ. Determinants of the signal averaged ECG after myocardial infarction: Relationship to infarct size and site in an experimental canine model. PACE 12:665, 1989.

9. El-Sherif N, Turitto G. High Resolution Electrocardiography. Futura Publishing Company, Inc., Mt. Kisco, NY, pp 279-298, 1991.

10. Gardner PI, Ursell PC, Fenoglio JJ, Wit AL. Electrophysiologic and anatomic basis for fractionated electrograms recorded from healed myocardial infarcts. Circulation 72:596-611, 1985.

11. Vaitkus PT, Kindwall KE, Marchlinski FE, Miller JM, Buxton AE, Josephson ME. Differences in electrophysiological substrate in patients with coronary artery disease and cardiac arrest or ventricular tachycardia. Circulation 84:672-678, 1991.

12. Schwarzmaier H-J, Karbenn U, Borggrefe M, Ostermeyer J, Breithardt G, Balkinhoff K. Relation between ventricular late endocardial activity during intraoperative endocardial mapping and low-amplitude signals within the terminal QRS complex on the signal-averaged surface electrocardiogram. Am J Cardiol 66:308-314, 1990.

13. Vassallo JA, Cassidy D, Simson MB, Buxton AE, Marchlinski FE, Josephson ME. Relation of late potentials to site of origin of ventricular tachycardia associated with coronary heart disease. Am J Cardiol 55:985-989, 1985.

14. Rozanski JJ, Mortara D, Meyerburg RJ, Castellanos A. Body surface detection of delayed depolarizations in patients with recurrent ventricular tachycardia and left ventricular aneurysm. Circulation 63:1172-1178, 1981.

15. Denniss AR, Johnson DC, Richards DA, Ross DL, Uther JB. Effect of excision of ventricular myocardium on delayed potentials detected by the signal-averaged electrocardiogram in patients with ventricular tachycardia. Am J Cardiol 59:591-595, 1987.
16. Dailey SM, Kay GN, Epstein AE, Plumb VJ. Modification of late potentials by intracoronary ethanol infusion. PACE 15:1646-1650, 1992.
17. Twidale N, Hazlitt HA, Berbari EJ, Beckman KJ, McClelland JH, Moulton KP, Prior MI, Lazzara R, Jackman WM. Late potentials are unaffected by radiofrequency catheter ablation in patients with ventricular tachycardia. PACE 17:157-165, 1994.
18. Marcus NH, Falcone RA, Harken AH, Josephson ME, Simson MB. Body surface late potentials: Effects of endocardial resection in patients with ventricular tachycardia. Circulation 70:632-637, 1984.
19. Hood MA, Pogwizd SM, Peirick J, Cain ME. Contribution of myocardium responsible for ventricular tachycardia to abnormalities detected by analysis of signal-averaged ECGs. Circulation 86:1888-1901, 1992.

3

Methods for Recording Late Potentials on the Body Surface

Electrograms shown in the previous chapter provided the direct evidence that depolarization of ventricular myocardium can outlast the surface-recorded QRS complex. These electrograms are in close proximity or even in direct contact with these late potential sources. Hence, these signals are of high enough amplitude (10–20 μV) that it is not difficult to record them with standard equipment. However, when body surface electrodes are used, these same signals are on the order of 1 to 10 μV and are not observable with standard ECG techniques. For example, the amplitude of a typical QRS complex is about 1.0 μV, hence a body surface late potential may be 1000 times smaller than the QRS complex. The primary use of the high-resolution ECG is to noninvasively record these low-level cardiac late potentials. A number of issues are involved in obtaining these recordings. Some of these include parameters that are historically based and do not necessarily provide us with any sense of optimization. Other issues are also highly technical. The goal of this chapter is to break down the SAECG procedure into its individual components and point out not only the current approach, but also to give a rationale for each component. Thus, as the techniques for recording of cardiac late potentials evolve, one may be able to understand the basis of the improvement. Several reviews and general reports provide the background for this section.[1-6]

Lead Systems

SAECG acquisition and analysis are based on the recording of three leads in an anatomically orthogonal configuration and are referred to as XYZ leads, similar to the coordinate axes used in geometry. The question often arises as to why these three leads are used. Frankly, the answer is most likely based on the fact that technology used by early investigators was limited in the number of low-noise amplifiers available and the relatively slow speed of the computers. For example, three leads would require only 25% of the computing time if one performed an SAECG on all 12 leads of the standard ECG. Since the early workers had to limit the number of leads to be analyzed, the XYZ set seemed to be a reasonable compromise from both a computing standpoint and a biophysical standpoint. Orthogonal leads formed the basis of vectorcardiography, which was popularized in the 1950s. It was thought that all of the electrical information generated by the heart could be represented by as few as three leads. Schemes were developed to derive an optimal set of three leads by using multiple electrode sites combined into a single lead. These so-called "corrected" orthogonal leads were aimed at creating a truly orthogonal lead set, independent of body shape. The most notable of these systems is the Frank lead system, which uses a resistor weighing network and an extra lead position to form its XYZ lead set. The practice in SAECG, however, is to use an uncorrected bipolar lead set. Figure 3.1 shows an idealized male torso with the seven electrode sites forming the XYZ lead set and a reference electrode. Note that the reason for using these sites is because of the early limitations in recording technology. Also, these lead positions were not optimized for identifying sites of the largest amplitude late potential activity.

The anatomic landmarks for positioning the electrodes are as follows. The X axis is from side to side. The X+ lead is placed along the left midaxillary line at the level of the fourth intercostal space. The X– lead is also placed at this level, but along the right midaxillary line. The Z+ lead is at the same level as the X lead and is placed on the anterior chest along the midclavicular line. The Z– is placed on the reflection of the Z+ electrode on the patient's back. Note that this differs from traditional vector cardiography where the positive Z electrode was on the back. The Y+ lead is placed on the lower torso also along the left midclavicular line. One standard says this can be on the left iliac crest, or even on the left leg.[3] The problem with the latter position is that one should avoid large muscle masses because they are a major source of noise due to their EMG signals. The Y– lead is usually placed in the suprasternal notch. In some earlier studies it was also placed in the subclavicular space along the same line as the Y+ and Z+ leads. The consensus is that it be placed in the

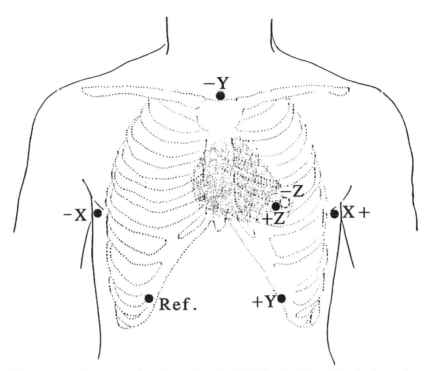

Figure 3.1. Anatomic locations for the XYZ leads. The X lead electrodes are lateral along the midaxillary line at the level of the fourth intercostal space. The X+ lead is on the left side. The vertical Y lead has electrodes at the xiphoid process (Y–) and the lower left abdominal quadrant (Y+). The Z+ electrode is at the same level as the X lead along the midclavicular line and the Z– electrode is the reflection of the Z+ on the back. (Reprinted with permission of the American Medical Association, Arch Intern Med, 148:1859-1863, 1988.)

suprasternal notch. The site marked "Ref." in Figure 3.1 is similar in function as the right leg electrode used in 12-lead ECG systems. It is shown in the lower right abdominal quadrant but its exact position is not critical since its only purpose is to provide a common reference point for the other leads. In some systems it may be a "driven" ground, which helps reduce overall noise in all leads.

As more knowledge is gained about the distribution of late potentials on the body surface, this XYZ lead set may be modified in the future. In particular, more lead sites placed nearer to specific infarct regions may eventually augment these original lead positions. This is particularly true since the technical reasons for using a limited lead set are no longer present with the advent of faster and cheaper microprocessors used in the commercial SAECG systems.

A practical, yet very important, consideration for obtaining a high-quality SAECG is the attention given to skin preparation when affixing the electrodes. Experience has shown that skin abrasion and alcohol cleaning prior to the electrode placement on the skin will significantly lower the noise, particularly any 60 Hz interference that may be present. There has been no systematic study of specific electrode types currently in use for several ECG applications and therefore none have been demonstrated to be superior. However, as an SAECG may take between 5 and 20 minutes for data acquisition, stable self-adhesive electrodes should be used. The reason for this is that a high-quality biophysical amplifier requires a balanced input impedance in order to reject the maximum amount of 60-Hz interference. For this same reason, an unbalanced input impedance as used in the Frank lead systems with its resistor weighing network may cause problems in some systems. In addition, a mechanically stable electrode-skin interface will limit noise because the electrochemical potentials at the interface will be minimized.

Instrumentation

Early studies relied on custom-built systems for recording the SAECG. Today, there are several commercial systems for recording the SAECG. In discussing the hardware, no single system will be described, but a more generic approach will be taken. In general, the hardware requirements are not technically demanding, but certain minimum specifications should be met. Figure 3.2 is a block diagram of a generic SAECG system and will be used to develop the description of the "typical" system.

Once the ECG leads are properly located and affixed, these XYZ signals are directed to low-noise biophysical amplifiers. The key features of these amplifiers are that they meet the standards for leakage current and patient isolation, and they must be defibrillation protected. Because these amplifiers are differential, they must be able to limit 60-Hz electrical line interference, which is often electrostatically coupled into the system. Such amplifiers are said to have a high common mode rejection. The gain of the amplifier should be as high as possible without exceeding the range of the analog-to-digital converter. In other words, it is important that the full amplitude of the QRS be maintained, without distortion, while fully digitizing signals 1000 times smaller.

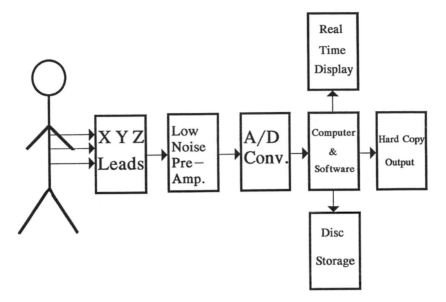

Figure 3.2. The general block diagram of the hardware used to acquire the SAECG. In most cases today, these elements are embedded within a 12-lead ECG system.

There are several types of filters used in obtaining an SAECG. Some of these filters are built into the instrumentation with electronic components and are referred to as analog filters. Other types of filters are implemented with computer algorithms and operate on the signals after they are digitized. They are called digital filters. Both analog and digital filters can perform the functions of high-pass, low-pass, and bandpass filtering. A high-pass filter will pass all signals above a specified frequency and attenuate signals below this frequency. The low-pass filter performs the opposite function and will pass signals below a specified frequency and attenuate signals above this frequency. Figure 3.3 shows a graph representing signal amplitude as function of frequency. The values of the curve are the relative amplitude of the output signal at each given frequency. The left side of the curve is where the filter is performing the high-pass function and the right side of the curve is where the filter is performing the low-pass function. Taken together they form a bandpass filter. The frequency axis has two specific frequencies marked at 0.05 Hz. and 300 Hz. When projected up to the actual graph, they indicate points that are about 70% of the flat part of the curve. They are often referred to as "corner frequencies" because

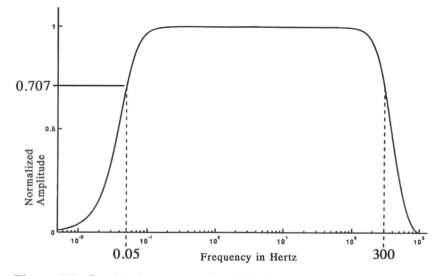

Figure 3.3. Graphical representation of the frequency response of a band-pass filter. The graph depicts the amplitude ratio of the output to input signals (vertical axis) of a bandpass filter as a function of frequency (horizontal axis). The frequency axis is logarithmic. This particular filter shows that the output signals are about 70% of the input signals at 0.05 Hz and 300 Hz. These are the high-pass and low-pass corner frequencies, respectively.

they are at the curved part of the graph. The vertical amplitude axis is normalized to 1, which means that a signal into the filter should not change its amplitude at frequencies where the amplitude is 1. The frequency axis of this graph is on a logarithmic scale to allow the display to cover several orders of magnitude. Note that at frequencies between the high-pass corner frequency of 0.05 Hz and 300 Hz, the curve is essentially flat and at a value of 1. This is the pass band of the filter and implies that these frequencies go through the filter unchanged. The curve on either side of the corner frequencies tapers down with a slope, on a logarithmic scale of 20 dB/decade. The dB unit is for decibels where the 70% value is about 3 dB. The decade represents the power of 10 change of the frequency scale. For example, 0.1 to 1.0 Hz is a decade as is 100 to 1000 Hz. The slope of the amplitude versus frequency curve is a figure of merit for most filters. The steeper the curve, e.g., 20, 40, or 60 dB/decade, the lower the amplitude of the frequencies outside the pass band. This discussion of filters has focused on the amplitude response of a filter. Equally important is the phase response of the filter which relates the timing or phase shift introduced by the filter at each frequency. The phase response curve is nonlinear for analog filters and those digital filters designed to mimic analog filters. A discussion of phase response, as it applies to the digital filters used in late potential detection, will be presented in Chapter 4.

At this point, the discussion of filters will be limited to the analog filters typically used in the electronic front end of the SAECG system. In effect, these filters provide a wider bandwidth than is required for the standard ECG. The use of digital filters that are part of the SAECG analysis of late potentials is discussed in Chapter 4. However, the general principles of filtering discussed below also apply to the digital filters.

Limiting the frequency response is a common part of all instrumentation. In some cases such limitations are inherent to the system. For example, in older style electrocardiographs, ink pens or heat elements were on the ends of a mechanical stylus and the pens moved across the moving page of paper. Such devices cannot record in realtime high-frequency signals due to the mass and inertia of the mechanical system. In the design of the ECG amplifier, it is not practical to have the amplifiers respond to direct current or to very low-frequency signals because they may be of significant magnitude, and the amplification necesssary for the ECG level signals would cause these low-frequency signals to overwhelm or saturate the amplifier so that the signals are out of the range of the system. These low-frequency signals are often seen as baseline wander on an ECG. The cause of such noise is usually a poor skin-electrode interface and often will resolve in a few minutes as the electrochemical reaction at the skin-electrolyte-electrode interface reaches an equilibrium. Standard ECG settings for the high-pass filter are 0.05 Hz and will limit, but not eliminate, this form of interference. Some of the commercial systems (primarily those with a 12-lead ECG function) use digital algorithms to limit this type of noise. It is still good practice to use traditional electronic filters for the initial high-pass filter function.

Typical ECG systems will use a low-pass analog filter in the range of 100 to150 Hz, but because of the higher frequencies in the SAECG, a low-pass filter of 300 Hz is the norm. This frequency represents a compromise between a requirement for the high-resolution ECG to have high fidelity while minimizing the noise. It is very important, in systems that digitize real-world signals such as the ECG, that there be some form of low-pass filter to limit a phenomenon known as aliasing. This phenomenon occurs when signals have frequencies greater than 50% of the digitizing rate. In such cases there can be an artifact whereby these higher frequencies "fold back" and appear as lower frequencies, even to the point of negative frequencies. Most people have seen such effects in old Western movies whereby the film speed of the camera cannot "digitize" the rotation of the wagon wheels and they sometimes appear to be going backwards. For practical purposes, the 300-Hz low-pass frequency is more than adequate for the SAECG. In Holter systems where there is a poor bandwidth at the higher frequencies, caution should be used when these systems are used for late potential analysis. A frequency response less than 100 Hz may unduly distort, in a nonsystematic fashion, the late potential parameters.[7]

Data Acquisition

Once we are sure that there are high-quality signals, the next step in the SAECG process is to convert these real-world, time-varying ECG voltages to the digital domain of the computer. The device for performing this task is aptly named an analog-to-digital converter (A/D converter or ADC). These devices will measure the voltage on a fixed time interval basis. This is known as the sampling frequency. In the SAECG systems, this is usually 1000 or 2000 times per second for each of the XYZ leads. At each tick of the digital clock, a number is generated that is transferred to the computer. The accuracy of this number depends on the number of levels or steps the ADC has between its voltage extremes. Figure 3.4 shows a stylized QRS complex in the upper left-hand corner. The ADC is depicted as a sampler and digitizer. The differences in sampling rate and digitizing resolution are shown in the two digitized QRS complexes below the original QRS. The middle QRS has an almost skyline appearance. There are large jumps in the signal character, both horizontally (low time sampling rate) and vertically (low resolution of digitizer). The bottom QRS improves in both of these aspects where the apparent sampling rate is faster and the digital resolution is greater. This signal still has a staircase appearance but more closely resembles the original QRS. In a good digital system, there should be no visual remnants of the digitizing process. A typical ADC for SAECG analysis will sample with a minimum of 1000 Hz (1 msec between sample points) and resolve in the amplitude at least 1 part in 4000. Technically, this is a 12-bit ADC. Several systems have used 16 bits of vertical resolution, which is 1 part in 65,000. While the 16-bit resolution is clearly superior, there is little difference in these systems from a clinical diagnostic perspective.

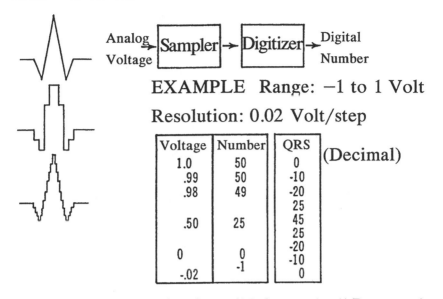

EXAMPLE Range: −1 to 1 Volt

Resolution: 0.02 Volt/step

Voltage	Number	QRS
1.0	50	0
.99	50	-10
.98	49	-20
		25
.50	25	45
		25
0	0	-20
	-1	-10
-.02		0

(Decimal)

Figure 3.4. The process of analog to digital conversion (A/D converter). The upper right section of this figure shows the steps between an analog voltage and a digital number—the process of analog to digital conversion. The first step is the sampler, which "holds" the analog signal for a short period of time while the digitizer "converts" this voltage to a digital number. The chart on the bottom right lists the voltage and its respective number produced by the A/D converter for the example QRS. In this case the resolution is given as 0.02 V/step. Hence a voltage of 1.00 and 0.99 V has the same level output of 50. The figures on the left represent the smooth analog voltage (*top*) and the effects that poor resolution digitizing would have on the digitized waveform (*middle*). The higher sampling rate and more levels of resolution result in less of "skyline" appearance (*bottom*).

Signal Averaging

As the ECG signals are being stored in the computer, several steps in the computer software are used to perform the actual signal average. We will try to break these into salient components, but before proceeding with this discussion, a few simple diagrams may aid in visualizing this process.

Figure 3.5 shows a simple representation of an ECG rhythm strip across the top. The stylized QRS complexes are labeled 1, 2, 3,...N, where the three dots represent an ongoing repeating rhythm. The first function of the computer program is to detect and align each QRS complex in the computer memory. This is depicted by the vertical alignment of the QRS complex along the left side of the

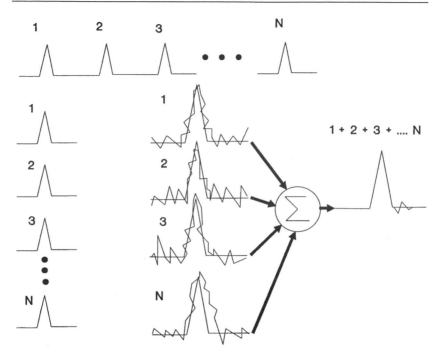

Figure 3.5. Diagrammatic representation of signal averaging. The top row represents a sequence of QRS complexes. The signal-averaging process must identify each QRS complex, shown vertically aligned on the left side. These same complexes are shown amplified with superimposed exaggerated noise signals. On a point-by-point basis, these signals are summated yielding a relatively noise-free signal.

figure. Next to each beat is an enlarged version of the QRS with an exaggerated noise signal drawn over each complex. As each is detected and aligned, the signals are summated on a point-by-point basis. This is represented by the circle with the summation symbol, Σ. The low noise output is shown as the output of the summation and has a small post-QRS potential or late potential. This brief explanation of signal averaging should aid the reader as a reference for the following discussion.

Beat Detection and Alignment

The first step in implementing the SAECG software is the detection and alignment of the QRS complexes. In some systems this is a completely transparent process for the user, while in others it is possible to tune the process to enable greater accuracy and flexibility in signal averaging, examples of which will be given below. Detecting QRS complexes by the computer is rather straightforward because it is the component of the ECG with both the largest amplitude and the most rapidly changing signal. However, just detecting large, rapidly changing voltages means that all QRS complexes, including premature ventricular beats, and artifacts will also be detected. Thus the second step in the process is QRS selection based on morphological or shape considerations.

Figure 3.6 shows a rhythm strip in the top tracing of several normal sinus beats and a premature ventricular contraction. Note the dotted line across the top could be used to show where the QRS detector might choose to identify each QRS complex if amplitude is the only detection criterion. In this case it would also detect the premature ventricular contraction. This initial detection point could be based on reaching a predetermined threshold level of the QRS itself. In addition to detecting premature ventricular contractions, this approach would also be susceptible to incorrectly detecting large T-waves such as those seen in hyperkalemia. Often, the time derivative of the QRS is used because the rate of change in ECG voltage is typically greatest during the QRS complex. In either case, this initial detection point is often referred to as the fiducial point within the QRS because it acts as a time reference for other operations in the QRS detection/alignment process. This point is shown in the middle panel of Figure 3.6. Neither the QRS amplitude nor the amplitude of the derivative of the QRS will provide an accurate enough fiducial point for signal averaging. By considering the shape of the QRS, one can accomplish two things. The first is a more accurate detection of the QRS by eliminating premature ventricular contractions, excessively noisy beats, and motion artifacts. The second advantage for using QRS shape is to allow the system to finely align each QRS complex for purposes of averaging.

The most common method to incorporate the shape of QRS is correlation. This process compares each incoming beat with a preselected template beat. In some commercial systems the user will select the template, while in others the computer will choose the template. In some cases the template is an average beat from the first 10 seconds of signal acquisition or it can be changed dynamically and be based on the signal average itself after the first 10 or 20 beats are averaged. This initial part of the signal averaging process could be considered a learning phase. If the template is automatically chosen, the learning process must be understood in order to avoid cases where premature ventricular contractions maybe included in

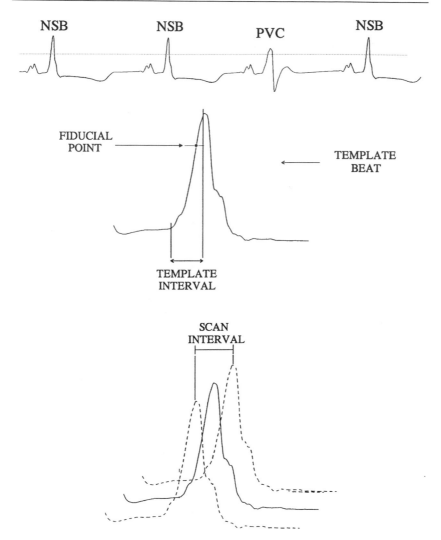

Figure 3.6. The process of correlation used to classify beats. The top trace shows three normal sinus beats (NSB) and a single premature ventricular contraction (PVC). A simple amplitude detector, depicted by the dotted line, would not discriminate between the NSB and PVC complexes. A template beat, or typical beat, is selected by the user or a software algorithm and all succeeding beats are compared by correlation. Correlation takes place over a portion of the QRS complex called the template interval. The fiducial point represents the center of this template interval and is chosen by the software. Each incoming beat "slides" across the template with a correlation coefficient value calculated at each point. The maximum value of the correlation coeffi- cient must exceed a predetermined threshold value for the beat to be included in the average. It also serves as the means of alignment for averaging.

the template learning process. Depending on the patient's actual rhythm, this may or may not be a significant problem. For example, in the case of bigeminy where every other beat is a premature ventricular contraction then a template based on an average or median beat of the first 10 or 15 beats would not resemble either the sinus beat or the premature ventricular contraction and the averaging process will not progress.

In general, the entire QRS is not needed to form the actual template. This would require many unnecessary mathematical calculations during the detection and alignment process. A typical template interval is shown in the middle panel of Figure 3.6. In some systems it is possible to select the duration of the template and its position with respect to the fiducial point. An example where this flexibility has been useful is the analysis of P waves. In this case the template interval can be shifted to the P wave even though the fiducial point remains within the QRS complex.

Once the appropriate template is chosen, then each incoming beat can be correlated with this template. Correlation is a mathematical comparison of any two processes to determine their relatedness. Values can range between –1.0 and +1.0, where a value of 1.0 represents an exact match between the two processes. Depending on the processes, values greater than 0.8 can be considered a good match. Hence, it can be used to compare any number of measurements. Often it is used to compare the results of a new test, such as cardiac output using a radionuclide method, with the more established method, such as cardiac output measured using angiography. The latter is often referred to as the "gold standard." In the case of QRS detection and alignment, the template serves as the gold standard. Each incoming beat is compared to the template using the correlation formula. However, due to the beat-to-beat variation it is not always possible to perfectly align the new beat with the template and the incoming beat is compared repeatedly with the template in an incremental fashion. The incoming beat is scanned across the template by temporally shifting it and calculating the correlation coefficient for each shift. This results in a range of correlation values, and the time when the maximum occurs is considered the optimal alignment point for signal averaging. In applying the correlation technique to QRS complexes, it turns out that values greater than 0.95 are common and values of 0.99 and greater are not uncommon. It is surprising that many premature ventricular beats do not differ from sinus beats at correlation values in 0.9 to 0.95 range.

The bottom panel of Figure 3.6 shows how the incoming beat (dotted lines) is scanned across the template beat (solid line). The scan interval represents the number of correlations that are made for each new beat. The point in this interval that gives the highest correlation above a predetermined correlation coefficient threshold is used for beat alignment. If none of the correlation coefficients exceed this threshold, then the beat will be rejected and is not included in the average. Reasons for rejection could be excessively noisy beats, dissimilar QRS complexes, e.g., premature ventricular contractions, or artifacts.

Signal Averaging

Once the computer has detected and aligned a beat, it will be added on a point-by-point basis as part of the SAECG. This is done for each XYZ lead and this summated set of data is stored in the computer memory. Depending on the actual implementation, the computer may or may not divide the sum by the number of beats. Eventually, the sum must be divided by the number of beats added together in order to obtain a calibrated signal average. In some systems the division is performed at the time of signal analysis and display.

The time window over which the sum is performed and the sampling rate will determine the number of summations. For example, a 300-msec window that is sampled at 2000 Hz will yield 600 points per lead to be summed. Hence, there will be 1800 computer addition operations per beat accepted for averaging. As each beat is added the noise is reduced in the signal-average recordings. This is the primary reason for using the signal-averaging method because very low-level signals are usually masked in noise. Thus, standard ECG techniques are not adequate for recording these very low-level signals.

Theoretically the square root of the number of beats averaged will be the factor by which the noise is decreased. If 100 beats are averaged, then the noise will be reduced by a factor of 10. In practice this is only approximate because the characteristics of the noise may vary over time. The noise in the SAECG can originate from three sources. The first and probably most significant source of noise is the EMG signal generated by the skeletal muscles such as those in the chest wall. During normal physiological processes such as breathing, these muscles will generate signals that can interfere with low-level ECG signals. Other sources of noise are 60-Hz power line interference and electronic noise inherent in all electronic devices. The 60-Hz noise is best dealt with at the front end by having performed a good skin prep, using shielded cables, and avoiding proximity to electrical sources of 60 Hz, e.g., fluorescent lights, monitors, etc. Good amplifier design with modem electronic components is usually adequate for limiting inherent noise. Thus, the physiological source of noise is persistent and the primary reason why signal averaging is used.

Noise Calculations

When the SAECG was first developed, the number of beats included in an average was often based on a predetermined, fixed number of beats, e.g., 200 or 300 beats per average. This proved to be unsatisfactory because it was clear that each patient had specific noise and signal level characteristics. This focused attention on using some measure of noise reduction as a criterion for defining a valid low-noise signal average. There are several approaches used for measuring residual noise during signal averaging. Each method has its own rationale and it is often not possible to directly compare noise voltage values from the different methods. They can be shown to be mathematically or empirically related.

There are two noise measurement methods in use today. The first is a post-averaging method that examines the signal-averaged XYZ leads in a format known as the filtered vector magnitude. This signal is often abbreviated as fQRS. This signal is described in great detail in Chapter 4. Figure 3.7 shows four panels, each with a filtered vector magnitude recording. For purposes of this noise discussion, the filtered vector magnitude is a combination of the XYZ leads where the QRS complex is the large central waveform. The late potential region is shown by the late potential-labeled bracket. The period of interest for noise measurement follows the late potential region and is in the ST segment of the ECG. By choosing a region of this ST segment, one may assume that there is no cardiac signal present and one can average the value of a predetermined noise window, labeled in the figure. This value estimates the residual noise in the SAECG. Panel A is a single beat "average" and the noise level is quite prominent. Using the post-averaging method, a 100-msec window is demarcated and the root mean square value of this window is 4.75 μV. Similarly, the 10-beat (panel B) and 100-beat (panel C) averages have noise values of 3.11 μV and 0.76 μV, respectively. There are three disadvantages for calculating noise in this manner. First, this time window may also contain signal components and therefore the root mean square measurement is one of signal

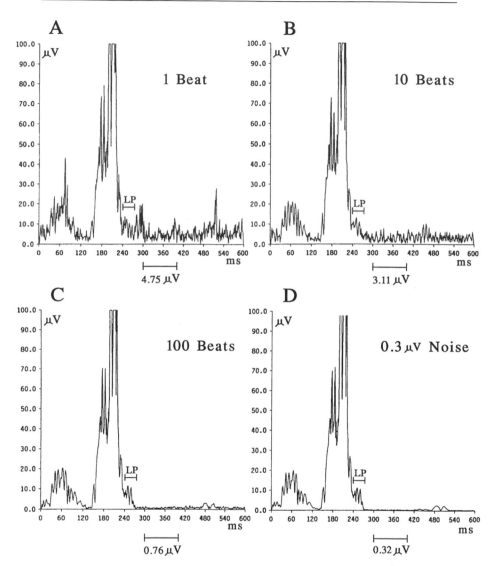

Figure 3.7. Examples of noise reduction as a function of the number of beats included in the average in the filtered vector magnitude recording. Panels **A**, **B**, and **C** show the filtered vector magnitude as after averaging 1, 10 and 100 beats, repectively. The late potential (LP) region is shown in panel. A noise value was calculated in a 100-msec window after the LP region. In panels **A**, **B**, and **C,** these noise values are 4.75 μV, 3.11 μV, and 0.76 μV, respectively. Panel **D** shows a signal that continued until this noise measurement decreased to 0.32 μV. Averaging to a preselected noise level rather than a fixed number of beats is the usual way used to terminate an average.

plus noise. Secondly, this value can be calculated only after the filtering and vector transformation has been performed and therefore is not a real-time method. Finally, the value that is calculated depends on the specific type and frequency setting of the high-pass filter. Several commercial systems use this approach and it was the method recommended in the Task Force Report. Frankly, it does not provide an accurate measure of noise, but if one uses a uniform approach to SAECG recording, it does allow a valid comparison. There are many ways to define noise so comparisons among various research reports and commercial systems are not usually directly comparable, although they may provide systematic or relative results. A 1.0-μV level on one system may be entirely different on another system.

Another method of noise calculation is based on the continuous measurement of the signal variance during the signal-averaging process. Each point in the SAECG waveform is an average and associated with each point is a variance and standard deviation. They are calculated in exactly the same manner as any statistical measure that uses the variance and standard deviation. In the field of statistical communications, the standard deviation is used as a direct measure of noise amplitude. Since the variance is just the square of the standard deviation, it is equated with the noise power. Hence, calculating the standard deviation during the signal-averaging process will yield a statistically valid measurement of the noise. It will also be independent of the amount of signal, if any is present. In the case of three XYZ leads with 600 points per lead, after each cardiac cycle, there would not only be 1800 average calculations but also 1800 standard deviation calculations. This is a large number of calculations for the computers used in typical SAECG systems. Selecting only a portion of the signal-averaging window for calculating the standard deviation will reduce the processing time and still provide valid estimates of the noise. This assumes that the noise does not change quickly over short periods of time, a property known as stationarity.

Each of the three leads of the SAECG may have a different noise level. One can combine the calculation of the standard deviation for each lead into a single noise figure during the averaging process. Thus, there is one noise figure that is calculated after each beat. If the noise is reduced by averaging the square root of the number of beats in the average, then the noise figure should reduce likewise. Figure 3.8 is a plot of the noise figure as a function of beats. Note that for the first 50 or so beats, the noise figure is somewhat variable.

NOISE FUNCTION
STANDARD DEVIATION

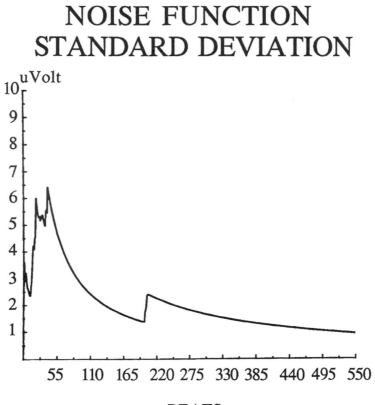

BEATS

Figure 3.8. This figure shows the level of noise as a function of beats in the average. This graph plots the noise calculated using the standard deviation method (see text) as beats are included in the average. During the initial 50 beats, the standard deviation values fluctuate and eventually decrease as a one over the square root of the number of beats. At about beat number 200 the subject raised his arms and then relaxed them. This is seen as a rapid increase in the noise level but then a return to the monotonic decline of the noise level. (Reprinted with permission of Futura Publishing Co.[1])

This is also true of the standard deviation calculation in general. After this initial variability the noise figure begins to decrease as predicted by signal averaging theory. To test the sensitivity of the noise factor, the test subject was asked to momentarily raise his arms, as if reading a book. This is seen in the noise function graph as an abrupt shift at about beat 190. Once the subject returned his arms to his side, the electromyographic noise returned to its basal state and the averaging process again began to diminish the noise, albeit from an offset due to the extra EMG activity.

The noise function can be used to quantify the noise for purposes of quality control. For example, if an average seems to take an excessively long time, one can examine the noise function to identify whether a relatively high noise was present throughout the averaging period or whether there were short bursts of noise. Such bursts can be caused by voluntary motion, e.g., body motion for position adjustment, or involuntary motion, e.g., coughing.

Another use of the noise function is to monitor noise during the averaging process and to use this as a decision tool for including or excluding beats from the average. While the correlation approach for beat selection and alignment works well for these purposes, it is not as well suited for noisy beat rejection. Hence, if the software calculates the noise function and detects a significant increase in noise based on some threshold change in the noise function, then the software can easily subtract out the beat that caused this shift. This becomes a quality assurance feature for the SAECG and is used in some fashion in most commercial systems.

Displaying, Printing, and Storing the Signal-Averaged Electrocardiogram

Once a high-quality SAECG is obtained, the system will make a set of measurements, described in detail in Chapter 4, and provide a printed page or hard copy of both the SAECG waveforms and these measurements. In some systems this printed information is the only permanent record of the SAECG results. Most of the systems sold today use a floppy disc to store the original data for later study or medical record archiving. These discs are usually compatible with most personal computers, and the vendors may provide software for further analysis and maintenance of a complete database. With the current state of digital technology, there are many approaches for performing these off-line forms of analysis. It is also possible to convert the SAECG files into formats acceptable by most vendors, thus allowing the digital exchange of SAECGs regardless of the make of the original acquisition system.

References

1. El-Sherif N, Turrito G (eds). High-Resolution Electrocardiography, Futura Publishing Co., Mt. Kisco, NY, 1992.

2. Gomes JA (ed). Signal Averaged Electrocardiography, Kluwer Academic Publisher, Dordrecht, Germany, 1993.
3. Breithardt G, Cain ME, El-Sherif N, Flowers N, Hombach V, Janse M, Simson MB, Steinbeck G. Standards for analysis of ventricular late potentials using high resolution or signal-averaged electrocardiography: A statement by a Task Force Committee between the European Society of Cardiology, the American Heart Association and the American College of Cardiology. Eur Heart J 12:473-480, 1991; Circulation 83:1481-1488, 1991, and Journal of the American College of Cardiology 17:999-1006, 1991.
4. Cain ME, Anderson JL, Arnsdorf MF, et al. American College of Cardiology Expert Consensus Document: Signal-averaged electrocardiography. J Am Coll Cardiol 27:238-249, 1996.
5. Technical Information Report of the SAECG Subcommittee of the American Association for the Advancement of Medical Instrumentation (AAMI). TIR-20:1999.
6. Lander P, Berbari EJ. Principles and signal processing techniques of the high-resolution electrocardiogram. Prog Cardiovasc Dis 35(3):169-188, 1992.
7. Berbari EJ, Rajagopalan CV, Lander P, Lazzara R. Changes in late potential measurements as a function of decreasing bandwidth. J Cardiovasc Electrophysiol 2:503-508, 1991.

4

Analyzing the Signal-
Averaged Electrocardiogram

Overview

The previous chapter focused on issues of SAECG acquisition, but this is just the first step in the overall process of obtaining an SAECG recording that identifies late potentials. After one is assured that a high-quality, low-noise SAECG has been obtained from the patient, the next step is the analysis of the SAECG. The primary waveform analyzed for cardiac late potentials is the filtered vector magnitude, as was shown in Figure 3.7. This signal is derived from the individual averaged XYZ leads. The derivation requires several signal-processing steps. Figure 4.1 summarizes these individual steps and shows the intermediate waveforms between the XYZ leads and the filtered vector magnitude.

Panel A in Figure 4.1 shows a 3-second rhythm strip of the individual XYZ leads at a typical amplitude and time scale that is familiar to the reader. Panel B has an expanded time scale (factor of 10) and amplitude scale (factor of 5) and shows the averaged QRS complex for each lead. Note that at the end of each QRS, several small deflections appear that are labeled as late potentials, but they are difficult to discern and quantify. Panel C shows each of these leads after processing with a high-pass filter implemented by the computer. The gain is further increased and the QRS complexes appear as rapid, multiple deflections, while the lower level terminal portions of the QRS complexes more clearly show the late potentials. As described in the previous chapter, a high-pass filter will attenuate signals below its corner frequency. The specific digital filters used in this process are discussed in greater detail in the next section. Panel D depicts the final step in deriving the waveform most commonly used in late potential analysis, the filtered vector magnitude,

41

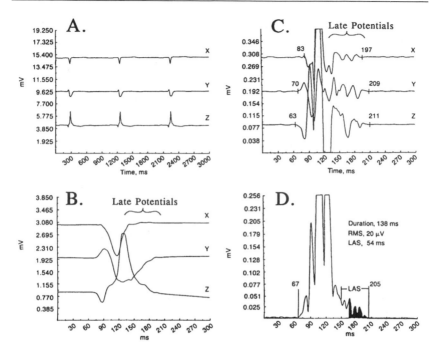

Figure 4.1. Visualization of the signal-averaging process and methods used to analyze the XYZ leads. Panel **A** is a 3-second rhythm strip of the XYZ leads. Panel **B** shows the signal-averaged XYZ leads in a 300-msec window. The gain is increased by a factor of 5 compared to panel **A**. There is a bracket identifying the late potential region after the QRS complex. Panel **C** shows the XYZ leads after filtering (40 Hz bidirectional, high pass) with the same late potential bracket. Panel **D** is the vector magnitude formed from the XYZ leads of panel **C**. The QRS duration is 138 msec; the darkened region is the RMS40 voltage measuring 20 μV; the low-amplitude signal (LAS) below 40 μV measures 54 msec in duration.

or fQRS. The fQRS is formed from the filtered XYZ leads using the formula from analytic geometry:

$$fQRS = \sqrt{X^2 + Y^2 + Z^2}$$

This results in a single waveform that has only positive values.

Two points are identified on the filtered vector magnitude. The first is the onset of the QRS complex, shown in panel D as a vertical line at 67 msec from the beginning of the averaging window. The second identification point is the QRS_{offset}, shown as a vertical line at 205 msec. These two points form the basis for three derived parameters: the QRS duration, or QRSd, the amplitude of the terminal 40 msec (RMS40 or V40), and the duration of the low-amplitude signal (LAS) below 40 μV. This overview provides an initial look at SAECG analysis. Following is an in-depth look at each individual step for deriving the filtered vector magnitude and the methods used to calculate its descriptive parameters.

Digital Filtering of the Signal-Averaged Electrocardiogram

Principles of filtering were discussed in Chapter 3, and in particular, the discussion focused on the traditional analog or electronically implemented filters. These are the filters built into the front-end instrumentation. This section will focus on digital filters that are implemented in computer software. These digital filters can perform many of the same functions as analog filters. Because the signals on which they operate are often stored in the computer, it is possible to perform filtering functions that are not possible with analog filters. This is the case with the most common digital filter used in analyzing the SAECG for late potentials. Before moving on to these specific digital filters, a short discussion of filter applications and signal composition follows. The practical knowledge of filters and signal manipulation will be useful in understanding the analysis of the SAECG.

The use of filters in the processing of electrical signals, including the SAECG, can be found in many ordinary, everyday devices. For example, the bass and treble controls on most stereo systems are a filtering technique to control the low-frequency and high-frequency components of the amplified signals, respectively. Sunglasses are optical filters aimed at reducing certain spectral components of light.

All signals can be represented as the sum of a set of constituent signals. The most common set of such a set of signals is sinusoids, i.e., sine and cosine functions. These oscillatory signals can be added together with each having a different amplitude, frequency, and phase. The left side of Figure 4.2 shows an example of four separate signals. Table 4.1 summarizes the relative characteristics of each signal.

Signal $X_1(t)$ is a constant or DC level with a relative amplitude of 1.0 having zero frequency and phase. Signal $X_2(t)$ is a cosine wave with a relative amplitude of 0.5, a frequency of 2 Hz, and a phase angle of 0°. Signals $X_3(t)$ and $X_4(t)$ have relative amplitudes of 1.0 and 0.67, respectively, and also phase angles of 0°. Their frequencies are 4 Hz and 6 Hz, respectively. The right side of Figure 4.2 is the

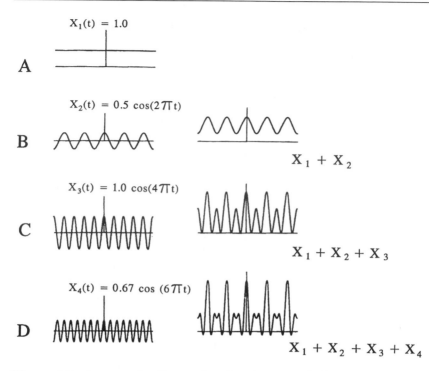

Figure 4.2. An example of a complex signal composed of a constant voltage (trace **A**) and three harmonically related cosine signals (traces **B**, **C**, and **D**). On the right side are three traces that show the sequential addition of the signals in traces **A-D**. The top right signal is the sum of trace A and B called $X_1(t)$ and $X_2(t)$, respectively. Similarly, the second and third signals on the right hand side are $X_1(t) + X_2(t) + X_3(t)$ and $X_1(t) + X_2(t) + X_3(t) + X_4(t)$, respectively.

Table 4.1
Oscillatory Signals and Their Characteristics

SIGNAL	Relative Amplitude	Frequency (Hertz)	Phase (degrees)
$X_1(t)$	1.0	0	0°
$X_2(t)$	0.5	2	0°
$X_3(t)$	1.0	4	0°
$X_4(t)$	0.67	6	0°

sequential sum of these signals. The top right signal is the sum of the DC level [$X_1(t)$] and the 2 Hz cosine wave [$X_2(t)$]. The middle signal is the sum $X_1(t) + X_2(t) + X_3(t)$. The bottom signal on the right side is the sum of all four signals. One can observe the emergence of a periodic signal, very similar to an ECG signal, with just the addition of these four signal components. In reality the standard ECG is a combination of an infinite number of sinusoidal signals between 0.05 and 150 Hz. Signals above and below these limits may be present in the ECG but they are not considered significant for the standard clinical uses of the ECG, e.g., the 12-lead ECG, the ambulatory ECG, the exercise ECG. The limits of 0.05 to 150 Hz are actually imposed by the filters (analog or digital) built into the ECG systems. In some cases the recording instrumentation does not extend even to these limits. Analog, tape-based Holter systems have a very poor low-frequency response and usually attenuate signals above 60 Hz.

Electronic circuits formed the initial methods of changing the frequency spectrum of signals and were discussed in Chapter 3. From the previous discussion it was noted that the hardware used to record the SAECG has a bandpass filter that passes all signals between 0.05 and 300 Hertz. Signals above and below these limits are attenuated at a predictable rate away from these two endpoints, as was depicted in Figure 3.3.

The Basics of Digital Filters

Once a waveform is digitized and stored in the computer, it ceases to be an actual voltage, but is represented as a series of numbers that are proportional to the voltages at the time they were actually sampled. These numbers can be manipulated as any other number and all of the standard arithmetic functions can be performed with the series of numbers representing an ECG. An example of a simple but highly useful digital filter is the derivative. The derivative of an analog waveform is the rate of change of the voltage versus time. This is written mathematically as dV/dt and signifies the change of voltage, dV, divided by the change in time, dt. The "d" operator before the voltage variable, V, and the time variable, t, are meant to represent an infinitesimally small change in either voltage or time. This concept of diminishing time is the basis of differential calculus. One need not become overly involved with these mathematical concepts of continuous time calculus because in the digital realm the difference in time is simply the sampling rate of the signal. For digital signals, the mathematical principles are based on discrete time intervals. The derivative is now the simple difference between adjacently sampled points and is more aptly expressed as $\Delta V/\Delta t$. Delta, Δ, is the change or subtracted difference between the two adjacent points. If the SAECG is sampled at 2000 Hz, then the $\Delta t = $ 0.5 msec.

Figure 4.3 is a graphical example of how the first difference, $\Delta V/\Delta t$, can be calculated for a time-varying SAECG recording of a single X lead. The adjacent points are subtracted in a pairwise fashion: point 1 minus point 2, point 2 minus point 3, etc. The inset of Figure 4.3 shows this graphically, where the small squares represent each digitally sampled point. The lower trace is the plot of the difference. Each point is equally spaced, and in order to calibrate the vertical scale, the difference in voltage is divided by a factor representing the sampling interval in seconds. The formula for this first difference is:

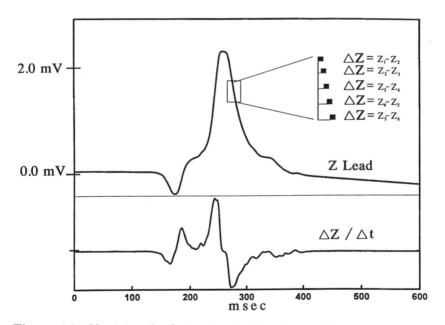

Figure 4.3. Obtaining the derivative of a digital signal. The top trace is a signal-averaged Z lead. The bottom trace is the first difference of this Z lead. On the top trace the rectangular box is blown up on the right to show individual data points, represented by the small solid squares. This demonstrates obtaining the sequential difference between adjacent points that are used to calculate the signal in the lower trace.

$$V_i = \frac{1}{K} (X_i - X_{i+1})$$

The variable, V, is the resulting first difference. The index, i, is used to count across both the output, V, and the original SAECG signal represented by X. The variable K is the proportionality constant for the time scale.

The first difference is a digital high-pass filter. If adjacent points are equal, regardless of their magnitude, the difference is zero. Thus, the first difference of slowly varying signals (or DC signals) will be small (or zero). The greater the difference between adjacent points the more rapidly the signal is changing in a given interval of time. This represents the high-frequency components of the signal. Thus, by attenuating low frequencies and preserving the higher frequencies the first difference is actually a high-pass filter.

If one were to add the values of two adjacent points instead of subtracting the values the resultant signal would be smoother version of the original. The smoothing filter is actually a low-pass filter. By including more than two points in this "moving average" the greater the smoothing function. It is common to average several points before and after the indexed value in the actual implementation. A 5-point smoothing function has the following formula:

$$V_i = \frac{1}{K} (X_{i-2} + X_{i-1} + X_i + X_{i+1} + X_{i+2})$$

The variables are the same as for the first difference equation, except that the output variable V is now the moving average. The moving average is the sum of five terms, the two prior to the index, i, the central point at i, and two points *after* the index. The scale factor K now includes a factor of five, representing the five points added, as well as the time scale. This moving average is a low-pass digital filter and demonstrates something not attainable with an electronic analog filter. An analog filter can only have an output based on the previous inputs whereas this digital low-pass filter function includes values that would be in the future (the i+1 and i+2 terms). Such a filter is physically unrealizable or noncausal in the analog domain. However, in the digital domain, the computer memory allows such filters to be implemented. This is a rather simple filter and is useful for demonstrating the power of digital filters. The recursion formula for more complex filters is beyond the intent of this book, but the most common digital filter used to analyze late potentials, the Simson bidirectional filter, is also a noncausal filter.

The Simson Bidirectional Filter

Dr. Michael Simson published the first clinically significant study of late potentials correlating their presence with ventricular tachycardia.[1] Among the several methodological steps was the bidirectional, high-pass filter. This filter used the digital implementation of the Butterworth filter. The Butterworth filter is a commonly used electronic filter that has what is called a maximally flat amplitude response, not unlike the one shown in Figure 3.3. The digital Butterworth filter is represented by a recursion formula that is a bit more complicated than those shown above for the first difference and moving average filter. Simson's contribution was to first apply this filter from the beginning of the averaging window to the mid-QRS region. The filter is then applied in reverse time order from the end of averaging window *backwards* to the same mid-QRS point. This is shown in Figure 4.4. The top trace is a signal-averaged lead. The bottom trace is the output of the Simson approach using a 40 Hz Butterworth filter. The fiducial or reference point marks where the filter changes its time sense. The signal to the left of the fiducial point is filtered in the normal or forward time sense. The computer reverses the time sequence in applying the same filter to the right of the fiducial point. Since the Butterworth filter can cause shifts in the timing of the signals, it became critical to limit these timing (phase) shifts that would occur at the end of the QRS. Hence the beginning and endpoints of the QRS shown at 63 msec and 211 msec, respectively, are not influenced by large signal components of the QRS complex. This results in minimal timing distortions at the endpoints. Signals before and after the QRS have the normal amount of phase distortion produced by the Butterworth filter, but this has not been considered a significant factor for late potential analysis. Note that the fiducial point, where the two filtering algorithms meet, produces a sharp deflection. This is an artifact of the bidirectional filter, and unless intra-QRS signals are of interest, it is of little consequence in standard late potential analysis.

The cardiac late potentials are very low-level signals normally masked by the QRS complex when they occur at the same time as the QRS complex. Regions of slow and/or delayed conduction may generate low-level depolarization potentials that occur well after the QRS complex. The use of a high-pass filter is aimed at limiting the

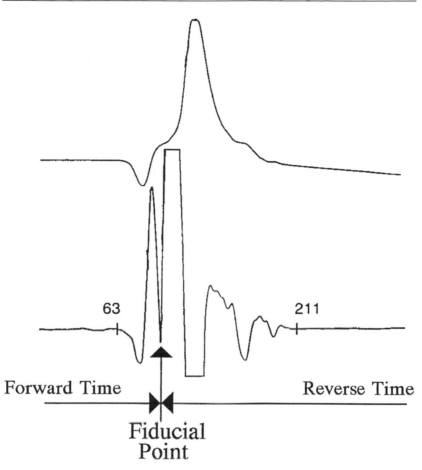

Figure 4.4. How the bidirectional processes a signal. The bidirectional filter uses the filter formula starting from both the left and the right side of the top signal, a signal-averaged Z lead. The fiducial point is in the mid-QRS region. The bottom trace is filtered output in the forward time sense from the left side and the reverse time sense from the right side.

amount of low-frequency energy in the terminal QRS complex and ST segment while preserving the amplitude of these higher frequency late potentials. The use of a standard analog or digitally implemented version of an analog filter will result in the shifting in time of some of the large QRS potentials into the period of the ST segment. This filtering artifact would mask the timing relationship of the late potentials (which are also shifted) with the QRS complex. The primary difficulty in dealing with these phase-shifted signals is that the amount of phase shift is *nonlinear* as a function of frequency. Hence the amount of phase shift is different for lower frequencies than it is for higher frequencies, and this could add an unaccountable timing discrepancy in late potential measurements. By applying the filter in a bidirectional fashion, the significant time shift of QRS energy is confined to the middle of the QRS complex and minimally distorts the timing relationship between the QRS endpoints and the late potentials. It was noted above that the late potentials have a higher frequency content than the QRS and ST segment. This assumption is discussed later in this chapter in the section on frequency domain analysis of the SAECG.

Parameters Derived from the Vector Magnitude

There are three parameters derived from the filtered vector magnitude. The first is the QRS duration, which is often abbreviated in the literature as fQRS or QRSd. The QRS duration is the difference between the end of the QRS (QRS_{offset}) and the beginning of the QRS (QRS_{onset}).

$$QRSd = QRS_{offset} - QRS_{onset}$$

In panel D of Figure 4.1, the QRSd is 138 msec. The QRS duration is a measure of total ventricular activation time; that is, it measures the time from the earliest ventricular activation to the time of latest ventricular activation. In the high-resolution mode, this applies to the termination of the low-level late potentials. The value of QRSd considered to be abnormal is variable among a number of studies depending on the study objectives, e.g., high specificity versus a high sensitivity. Abnormal QRSd values range from 110 to 120 msec, with the most common value being 120 msec. A systematic study of this variable is discussed later in the section on individual lead analysis.

The other two late potential parameters also rely primarily on the QRS_{offset} point. They are the root mean square (RMS) voltage and the low-amplitude signal (LAS) duration. Both are obtained from the filtered vector magnitude. They measure features of the late potential waveform and do not directly relate to the electrophysiology of the heart as the QRS duration does. Essentially, a late potential appears as a low-level "tail" after the main body of the QRS complex. The RMS and LAS are designed to be descriptors of this late potential tail. The threshold for an abnormal value of RMS40 is most commonly less than or equal to 20 mV, and for the LAS, values greater than or equal to 20 msec are considered abnormal.

Each measurement is discussed in greater detail below, but a common problem for interpreting these three parameters is how many of the parameters must be abnormal for the entire SAECG is considered abnormal. There is no straightforward answer and there is always a tradeoff between sensitivity and specificity. However, numerous studies have shown that the QRS duration is the most significant and commonly used parameter for analyzing the SAECG.

The QRS Duration

The initial animal studies that established late potentials as signals that are recordable from the body surface[2] compared their duration as measured from both the body surface and the epicardial surface. This study provided primarily qualitative data comparing signals from both types of recordings. However, this study did demonstrate that late potentials have concomitant heart rate-dependent changes when observed on both the body surface and the epicardial surface in the canine infarct model. A more systematic study by Simson et al.[3] in a similar canine infarction demonstrated a correlation coefficient of .93 between the two measures of late potentials. There were discrepancies where differences of 20–40 msec were observed in 15% of the cases. In each case the body surface measurement missed the detection of the full extent of the late potentials. A clinical study by Simson et al.[4] comparing endocardial catheter recordings with the SAECG demonstrated a correlative relationship between the QRS durations, but there were discrepancies as large as 60 msec.

A systematic study comparing the SAECG and electrogram measurements of late potential duration using the canine infarction model required three specific approaches to ensure a strong correlation.[5] The most significant approach was the use of the individual XYZ leads for determining the QRS_{offset} rather than the filtered vector magnitude. Another required approach was the use of an unfiltered, "normal" gain ECG for choosing the QRS_{onset}. And finally, due to the canine ECG characteristics, the Simson bidirectional filter was not used. Instead, a digital filter that exhibited very little phase shift was used because in the reverse time mode the Simson filter had problems with the dog's T wave producing overlapping signals with the late potentials. The use of individual leads in the clinical setting is discussed in the section on individual lead analysis.

The Root Mean Square Voltage

The shaded region of the filtered vector magnitude in panel D of Figure 4.1 depicts the last 40 msec of the QRS complex measured from the QRS_{offset}. The root mean square (RMS) voltage of this terminal 40 msec has a value of 20 mV. The RMS voltage of a signal can be considered an average voltage over a period of time. A true average of a time-varying voltage could be zero because sometimes the signal is positive and sometimes the signal is negative. For example, the average of a single period of a sine wave is zero because the signal has an equal set of positive and negative values. The RMS method squares each voltage value forcing all values to be positive, performs the average of these values, and then takes the square root of this average. Understanding this sequence of steps perhaps clarifies the term RMS. In some respects the RMS of the filtered vector magnitude is a bit redundant because it too was formed by squaring the signals and taking a square root.

The RMS is a voltage based on a time duration at the end of the QRS complex. This duration is usually 40 msec. At times this RMS parameter will be called RMS40 or V40 in the literature. A number of studies have suggested various values for an abnormal value for the RMS40. These range from 5 to 25 mV, with the most common value being 20 mV.

An RMS value can be calculated for each time window referenced to the QRS_{offset}. Thus, there are RMS values that range from the QRS_{offset} to the QRS_{onset}. This sequence of RMS values can be plotted and is shown in Figure 4.5. There is nothing particular to RMS40 and it appears as a single point in the RMS curve in Figure 4.5. This RMS function was studied in a series of patients to determine if one value was indeed optimal.[6] Panel A of Figure 4.6 shows the average of the RMS curves for two sets of patients. The first group is called the low arrhythmia risk group. These patients had electrophysiological studies for syncope evaluation but had no inducible or observed ventricular tachyarrhythmias. In addition, they had no prior infarct and had ejection fractions greater than 50%. The second

$\longrightarrow$

Figure 4.5. The root mean square (RMS) function. The top panel shows a filtered vector magnitude signal. The darkened region is the terminal 40 msec of this signal and its RMS value is calculated. By choosing every value from 0.0 msec (the QRS_{offset}) to the QRS_{onset} point will yield a plot shown in the lower trace. The actual mathematical formula for this curve is shown on the lower right. In this case the value of RMS40 can be read from the graph and is about 13 μV.

RMS TIME FUNCTION

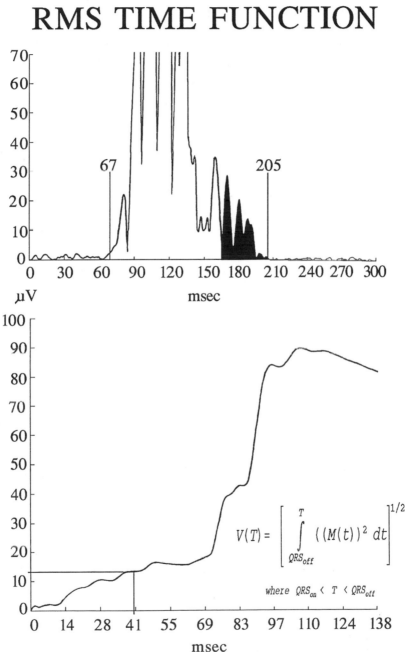

$$V(T) = \left[\int_{QRS_{off}}^{T} ((M(t))^2 \, dt \right]^{1/2}$$

where $QRS_{on} < T < QRS_{off}$

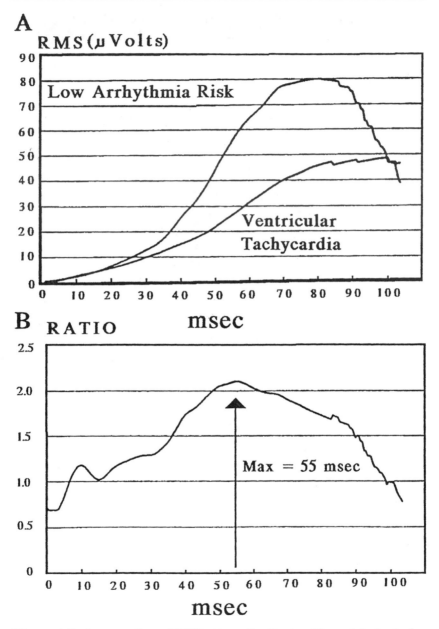

Figure 4.6. A comparison of RMS curves of patients with ventricular tachy-cardia and those with a low arrhythmia risk. Panel **A** shows an average of the RMS curves for both patient groups. The ratio of these curves is shown in panel **B**. The maximum value of the ratio occurs at 55 sec. (Reprinted with permission of the American Heart Association.[6])

group of patients had inducible ventricular tachycardia. The average plot for each group shows a clear separation. Panel B of Figure 4.6 shows the plot of the ratio of the two curves in panel A. The maximum of this ratio curve occurred at approximately 55 msec. This maximum ratio could be considered an optimal duration time for calculating the RMS function. However, reanalysis of the data using the value of RMS55 did not turn out to be a statistically better parameter than RMS40.

A conclusion reached by Lander et al.[6] concerning the RMS parameter is that it provides little incremental value to late potential analysis. Two other observations are important in arriving at this conclusion. The first is that the RMS parameter is strongly correlated with the QRS duration. Both measurements rely directly on the QRS_{offset} point. Second, small changes in the QRS_{offset} point, e.g., 1–5 msec, may change the QRS duration by a very small percentage, but the RMS40 could change by as much as 50%. These small changes in the QRS_{offset} point are usually due to low levels of residual noise still remaining after averaging. Hence the RMS40 parameter is very sensitive to residual noise while the QRS duration is a far more robust measurement.

Another conclusion from Lander et al.[6] is that an extremely small value of RMS40, i.e., below 4 mV or less, may point to an abnormal study. This result seemed to be independent of whether or not the QRS duration was abnormally long.

The Low-Amplitude Signal Duration

The low-amplitude signal (LAS) parameter is a duration based on a voltage measurement at the end of the QRS complex. A 40-mV voltage is the most commonly used reference point. In panel D of Figure 4.1 the LAS duration, using the 40-mV reference, is 54 msec. An LAS of greater than 20 msec is the most common definition of an abnormal LAS value. There have not been systematic studies of LAS to determine its sensitivity to residual noise as was the case for RMS. Since the LAS also relies directly on the QRS_{offset} point, it would also seem to imply that it too is correlated with the QRS duration measurement.

Individual Lead Analysis

As mentioned in the section on the QRS duration, there was an improved correlation between SAECG and epicardial measurement of QRS duration when the individual XYZ leads were used to measure the QRS duration. A theoretical study[7] showed that if each lead had a different signal-to-noise ratio, then the vector magnitude transformation would always have a signal-to-noise ratio that was lower than the highest individual lead signal-to-noise ratio. This study was followed by a clinical study comparing the QRS duration obtained from the vector magnitude with the longest QRS duration from the individual XYZ leads.[6] This resulted in an improved sensitivity with some loss in specificity. Rather than consider one approach over another, a nomogram was developed that considered both measurements of QRS duration. Figure 4.7 shows this graphical approach for interpreting the SAECG. It is based on a retrospective analysis and awaits full testing in a prospective study, but the approach has appeal since it now considers four possible clinical outcomes: normal, borderline normal, borderline abnormal, and abnormal. If one plots the QRS duration from the filtered vector magnitude (vertical axis) against the longest QRS duration from any of the XYZ leads (horizontal axis), the result will lie in one of these four regions. If the point lies in the upper left and lower right corners of the graph, the outcome is considered to be in error due to an algorithm problem or a technically poor study. In these cases the difference between the two QRS duration measurements is greater than 30 msec. If such errors occur, the study should be redone.

There are three steps that the user should follow prior to using the graph. If the standard ECG has a QRS duration of greater than or equal to 120 msec, the subject has either a bundle branch block or a severe intraventricular conduction defect. The use of the SAECG is contraindicated in such patients. The QRS_{offset} and QRS_{onset} should be checked for errors. The QRS_{onset} is most easily identified because it is usually derived from the standard or low-resolution ECG and requires the same skill as used in reading standard ECGs. Identifying the QRS_{offset} is bit more difficult. It requires visualizing and mentally estimating the residual noise level and whether or not the algorithm finds the end of the larger signal levels above this noise level. In most cases the algorithm is correct. In some cases where the human reader has difficulty with evaluating the correctness of the algorithm, the study can be repeated two or three times to allow the reader the opportunity to compare among them.

The third step prior to using the graph is to check the amplitude of the RMS40 parameter. As stated above, if this value is less than 4 mV, the study is considered abnormal.

1. If 12-lead ECG QRS duration is > 120 msec, SAECG cannot be analyzed by this method.

2. Check QRS onset and offset values for measurement error.

3. If the vector magnitude RMS40 is less than 4 mV, the SAECG is <u>abnormal</u>.

4. Otherwise, use the graph below:

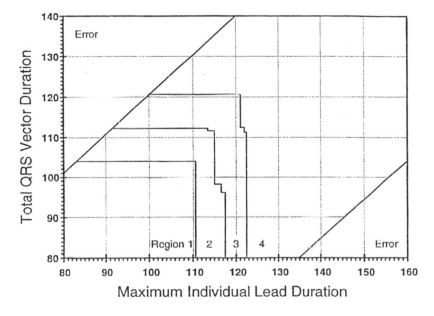

Region	Interpretation	Risk of serious ventricular arrhythmia
1	Normal	Very low.
2	Borderline normal	Low.
3	Borderline abnormal	Appreciable if accompanied by risk factors, such as reduced LV function, healed MI, spontaneous nonsustained VT.
4	Abnormal	Significant.
Error	Measurement error	Undefined.

Figure 4.7. A nomogram based on the QRS duration from individual XYZ leads and the filtered vector magnitude recordings. Items 1–4 lead the reader through several steps of which plotting the QRS durations is the final one. The nomogram is divided into four clinically interpretive regions: (1) normal, (2) borderline normal, (3) borderline abnormal, and (4) abnormal. Each region identifies a level of risk for serious ventricular arrhythmias from very low to significant. (Reprinted with perrmission of the American Heart Association.[6])

The four diagnostic regions relate the test result to the risk of a serious ventricular tachycardia. Region 1 is considered normal where the risk is very low. Here the vector magnitude QRS duration is below 104 msec and the longest duration QRS of either the X, Y, or Z lead is less than 111 msec. Region 2 is the borderline normal outcome and the arrhythmia risk is considered low. The vector magnitude QRS duration lies between 104 msec and 112 msec, and the longest duration QRS of either the X, Y, or Z lead is between 111 msec and 117.5 msec. Region 3 represents the patients who are the most problematic for the SAECG. In this region, the patients have an appreciable risk of ventricular tachycardia, but the note on the chart suggests that other clinical variables must be considered. This is of course true for the other regions as well, but particularly so for region 3. The vector magnitude QRS duration is between 112 and 121 msec while the individual lead is between 117.5 msec and 123 msec. Region 4 is the abnormal region where the patients have a significant risk of ventricular tachycardia. The fQRS duration is greater than 121 msec and the longest duration of the individual lead is greater than 123 msec. There are several places on the chart where the lines that separate the regions have a staircase feature so the times, listed above, that demark the regions are those on the coordinate axes. Each individual study should actually be plotted to account for these variations.

Frequency Domain Analysis

Thus far the entire emphasis of this book has been on the time domain analysis of the SAECG for detecting and quantifying late potentials. The analysis of the SAECG using frequency domain techniques has a strong rationale. The pathophysiological basis of late potentials is that there are viable regions within and surrounding an infarct that depolarize at times much later than they would have in a normal heart. Based on studies in canine infarction models, the pathways of conduction through these infarct regions may be slower and /or the pathways are longer due to circuitous pathways. In either case, the resulting extracellular electrograms usually exhibit a multiphasic character. In many cases these signals would outlast the normal duration QRS.

Analysis of ECGs for evidence of activation through diseased regions dates to studies by Langner in the 1950s[8] where the focus was on identifying slurs and notches in the QRS. Other studies by Flowers et al.[9] established that these high-frequency components of the QRS were correlated with varying degrees of heart disease that was quantified with postmortem studies. Other studies of the QRS complex for slurs and notches led to the scoring system of Selvester[10] and quantitative analysis by Goldberger et al.[11] Hence disruptions in the normal sequence of activation of the ventricles may be considered as macro-level events when they are visible in the standard ECG. When such events outlast the QRS, they usually reach the microvolt level and require the SAECG for recording and analysis. The character of these signals implies that they are fundamentally different from signals generated by normal myocardium and are activated in a normal sequence. These abnormal signals, either during or after the QRS, are postulated to have a different spectral composition than the normal ventricular signals. It is recognized that the disruption of the normal ventricular activation sequence may result in delayed activation of regions that are normally early in the QRS complex. Such delays may not outlast the QRS complex and are therefore not amenable to standard time domain analysis. Thus, frequency domain analysis would be one approach for identifying such abnormal, intra-QRS potentials. Unfortunately, the spectral resolution of frequency domain analysis does not provide an accurate means of separating the large-amplitude normal signals from the low-amplitude abnormal signals. Another approach, described in Chapter 8 , combines signal modeling and time domain analysis to separate these signal components, but it has not been widely tested in clinical practice.

The concept of sinusoidal composition of signals was introduced in Chapter 3 for the presentation of filtering theory. The signal-processing methods to analyze the various frequency components of a given signal are often limited when dealing with signals that change their character over a relatively short time period. For signals of limited time duration, the best one can do is estimate the spectral components, and a common tool for this is Fourier analysis, named for the French mathematician who first studied the analysis of heat transfer using spectral decomposition. The most common digital implementation is an optimized method called the fast Fourier transform (FFT). This is one of many approaches used to estimate the spectral composition of a signal.

The clinical use of spectral estimation methods for analyzing the SAECG is considered by most as an experimental approach. Initial clinical studies by Cain et al.[12] followed the strong rationale for spectral approaches as mentioned above but have relied on traditional Fourier methods that are not optimized for data windows as short as those encountered in SAECG work. This approach, along with a series of follow-up studies, has not been used widely in the clinical setting. An extension of the short-time FFT is the spectro-temporal approach[13] and the follow-up analysis of spectral turbulence.[14] For the most part, frequency domain analysis is still considered experimental and is not a primary focus of this book. The reader is referred to the above-referenced work for further details in spectral analysis of the SAECG.

References

1. Simson MB. Use of signals in the terminal QRS complex to identify patients with ventricular tachycardia after myocardial infarction. Circulation 64:235, 1981.
2. Berbari EJ, Scherlag BJ, Hope RR, Lazzara R. Recording from the body surface of arrhythmogenic ventricular activity during the ST segment. Am J Cardiol 41:697, 1978.
3. Simson MB, Euler D, Michelson EL, Falcone RA, Spear JF, Moore EN. Detection of delayed ventricular activation on the body surface in dogs. Am J Physiol 241:H363-H368, 1981.
4. Simson MB, Untereker WJ, Spielman SR, Horowitz LN, Marcus NH, Falcone RA, Harken AH, Josephson ME. Relation between late potentials on the body surface and directly recorded fragmented electrograms in patients with ventricular tachycardia. Am J Cardiol 51:105-112, 1983.
5. Berbari EJ, Lander P, Geselowitz DB, Scherlag BJ, Lazzara R. Identifying the end of ventricular activation: Body surface late potentials versus electrogram measurements in a canine infarction model. J Cardiovasc Electrophysiol 5(1):28-40, 1994.
6. Lander P, Berbari EJ, Rajagopalan CV, Vatterott P, Lazzara R. Critical analysis of the signal-averaged electrocardiogram: Improved identification of late potentials. Circulation 87:105-117, 1993.
7. Lander P, Deal RB, Berbari EJ. The analysis of ventricular late potentials using orthogonal recordings. IEEE Trans Biomed Eng 35:629-639, 1988.
8. Langner PH, Geselowitz DB, Mansure FT. High frequency components in the ECGs of normal subjects and of patients with coronary heart disease. Am Heart J 62:746, 1961.
9. Flowers NC, Horan LG. Diagnostic importance of QRS notching in high frequency electrocardiograms of living subjects with heart disease. Circulation 44:605, 1971.
10. Selvester RH, Wagner GS, Hindman NB. The Selvester QRS scoring system for estimating myocardial infarct size. Arch Intern Med 145:1877, 1985.
11. Goldberger AL, Bhargava V, Froelicher V, Covell J. Effect of myocardial infarction on high-frequency QRS potential. Circulation 64(1):34, 1981.
12. Cain, ME, Ambos HD, Witkowski FX, Sobel BE. Fast-Fourier transform analysis of signal-averaged electrocardiograms for identification of patients prone to sustained ventricular tachycardia. Circulation 69:711, 1984.

13. Haberl R, Jilge G, Pulter R, Steinbeck G. Comparison of frequency and time domain analysis of the signal averaged electrocardiogram in patients with ventricular tachycardia and coronary artery disease: Methodologic validation and clinical relevance. J Am Coll Cardiol 12:150-158, 1988.

14. Kelen GJ, Henkin R, Stares AM, Caref EB, Bloomfield D, El-Sherif N. Spectral turbulence analysis of the signal averaged electrocardiogram and its predictive accuracy for inducible sustained monomorphic ventricular tachycardia. Am J Cardiol 67:965-975, 1991.

5

The Normal Signal-Averaged Electrocardiogram, Technical Problems, Pitfalls, and Limitations

The Normal Signal-Averaged Electrocardiogram

The previous chapter emphasized how the SAECG is analyzed for identifying cardiac late potentials. There have been many SAECG studies of late potentials, but only a few have been devoted to identifying optimal values for defining the normal SAECG. Some studies have focused on healthy normal subjects in an attempt to define a normal SAECG, but this approach must viewed with caution. Extending a diagnostic test, originally designed to be used in a selected population, to normal subjects will most likely yield a significant number of false positives. Unless a very long-term follow-up is considered, then the use of the SAECG for late potentials should not be used in normal subjects. For example, cardiologists are aware of false positive problems associated with the exercise tolerance test and do not use it as a screening test for the general population. Similar caution is advised for use of the SAECG and it should not be considered as a screening test in the general population.

The values of the SAECG parameters used to separate normal and abnormal have been based on many studies, but most of these were not based on a large number of patients. In addition, the use of an abrupt threshold, e.g., QRS duration (QRSd) >120 msec, is not a common practice for other continuous variables in medicine. The literature is not strong in recommending whether one, two, or three of the standard SAECG variables must be in the abnormal range. Most of the multiparameter studies that have examined the risks of future ventricular tachyarrhythmias have shown that the QRSd variable is independent and the most significant late potential measurement. However, many practitioners will require one of the three late potential measures to be abnormal to define an abnormal study. The graph shown in Figure 4.7 demonstrated an approach that considers primarily the duration in the filtered QRS and the longest duration in an individual XYZ lead. This approach refines the outcome to consider the borderline cases and was discussed in more detail in Chapter 4.

A question that may arise in the analysis of the SAECG is whether the relative change in the QRSd is more important than its absolute value. Consider the patient with a QRSd of 110 msec as measured on the standard 12-lead ECG. For the sake of argument, consider that this patient does not have any form of bundle branch block. Suppose the SAECG from this hypothetical patient has a QRSd of 115 msec, which is considered in the abnormal range at many centers. Does this 5-msec difference between two methods of QRSd measurement constitute an abnormal finding? Now consider the following patient with a QRSd of 80 msec on the 12-lead ECG and a QRSd of 110 msec on the SAECG. This latter value is considered normal at most centers. Does the 30-msec difference between the two measurements constitute a significant clinical observation? In the first case the difference may be due more to an improved resolution in measuring the depolarization time of normal myocardium, while in the second case there is clearly a low-level signal that far outlasts normal myocardial depolarization. Unfortunately there have been no clinical studies that have investigated these types of questions. A study by Okin et al.[1] examined the absolute difference between the standard 12-lead QRSd and the longest QRSd in any of the signal-averaged XYZ leads. They demonstrated an improved specificity from 79%, using the standard late potential measures, to 89% using a regression analysis of the absolute difference. The sensitivity in this case was relatively unchanged. The regression analysis found an inverse relationship between the absolute difference and the QRSd of the SAECG. That is, as the standard ECG measure of the QRSd increased, a shorter difference between the two QRSd measurements was required for a positive test.

There are several factors that may directly influence the interpretation of the SAECG, particularly the QRSd, since these factors are known to alter the QRSd of the standard ECG. Specifically, the role of gender and age are known to influence the QRSd as measured in the standard ECG. It is known that the QRSd of normal females, as measured on the standard 12-lead ECG, is about 8 msec shorter than the similarly measured QRSd of normal males.[2] A few reports utilizing the SAECG have also compared the QRSd of males and females[3,4] and showed that there is indeed a 7-10 msec difference in separating low risk and high risk male and female patients. This reported difference between males and females has not been widely used in defining an abnormal SAECG.

Aging also affects the QRSd of the standard ECG. In this case there is an inverse relationship where the QRSd is longer in younger people than in older people.[5] The average QRSd for males between 18 and 29 years is 96.4 ± 8.6 msec, and for males at age 50, the average QRSd is 92.7 ± 9.3 msec. For females, the role of aging is negligible on the duration of the QRS complex. While the gender-related differences in the standard QRSd translated to the SAECG, it is not clear what role aging has on the SAECG measures of the QRSd of adults. In one study, age-related criteria were developed for the pediatric population.[6]

The role of age and gender in SAECG interpretation was a focus in the largest multicenter, multivariate study of late potentials following myocardial infarction.[7] This report was part of the CAMI (Canadian Assessment of Myocardial Infarction) study and collected data from 2461 patients without bundle branch block from nine institutions. This large study reaffirmed the primary value of the QRSd parameter over the RMS or LAS parameters as being an independent marker for arrhythmia risk. Gender, age, and infarct location also significantly influenced the interpretation of the SAECG. The investigators found shorter QRSd values in females, divided the patients into four age groups (<50 , 50 to 59, 60 to 69, and 70 to 75 years of age) and two infarct locations (non-Q wave + inferoposterior versus anterior).

The Role of Filtering in Late Potential Identification

The use of both analog filters and digital filters has been discussed in the context of data acquisition and analysis. The analog low-pass filter is used prior to digitization to limit aliasing, the phenomenon where higher frequencies can appear as lower frequencies due to low sampling rate. Digital high-pass filtering is used to separate low-frequency signals in the ST segment from the lower amplitude late potentials. However, there many options associated with the high-pass filter that can significantly change the interpretation of the SAECG. The type of high-pass filter most commonly used in the analysis of late potentials is the original bidirectional filter described by Simson.[8] There are many variables when actually implementing the filter that can markedly change the interpretation of the SAECG. These include the corner frequency and the filter order. One study demonstrated the changes in sensitivity and specificity based on the cutoff frequency of the high-pass filter[9] and showed that a 25-Hz filter produced results with the lowest sensitivity (compared to the other cutoff frequencies) while the 80-Hz filter produced results with the highest specificity. The 40-Hz filter produced intermediate values for both sensitivity and specificity.

Figure 5.1 shows the changes in the XYZ leads (right side) and the filtered vector magnitude (left side) as a function of the high-pass corner frequency using the Simson approach of bidirectional high-pass filtering with corner frequencies of 25 Hz, 40 Hz, and 80 Hz. All data are from the same patient. The QRSd in panels A, B, and C are 142 msec, 114 msec, and 105 msec, respectively. Hence, this subject's QRSd ranges from an abnormal value to a borderline value to a normal value strictly as a function of the filtering process. On the right side, the individual XYZ leads show a range of values for the QRSd, also as a function of filtering. In practice, the 80-Hz range is seldom used, and the most commonly reported value of the high-pass corner frequency is 40 Hz. Note that in Figure 5.1, the QRSd of the individual XYZ leads all have values greater than 130 msec, while the QRSd of the filtered vector magnitude is 114 msec. These data support analysis of the individual leads as put forth in Chapter 4.

There has been interest in observing late potentials from the tape-recorded ambulatory (Holter) ECG. There are several precautions that one must have with the analog tape-based recorders due to their inherently low-frequency response. Most analog tape-based systems have a high-frequency response well below 100 Hz and may be as low as 25 Hz[10] so in general they are not adequate for full-fidelity recordings of late potentials. The role of the low-pass filter cutoff frequency was systematically studied in a group of 75 patients, half of whom had late potentials and ventricular tachycardia, while the other half had no late potentials or inducible ventricular tachycardia.[11] Hence, this group started with 100% sensitivity and specificity. Figure 5.2 is an example of how the QRS_{offset} and QRS_{onset} points both vary as a function of the low-pass filter frequency. All of the filtered vector magnitude waveforms in Figure 5.2 are from the same data file. At cutoff frequencies below 100, the QRS_{onset} point changes as much as 20 msec. The QRS_{offset} point changes more than 30 msec when the cutoff frequency is below 100 Hz. Thus, systems with a

VECTOR MAGNITUDE   X Y Z LEADS

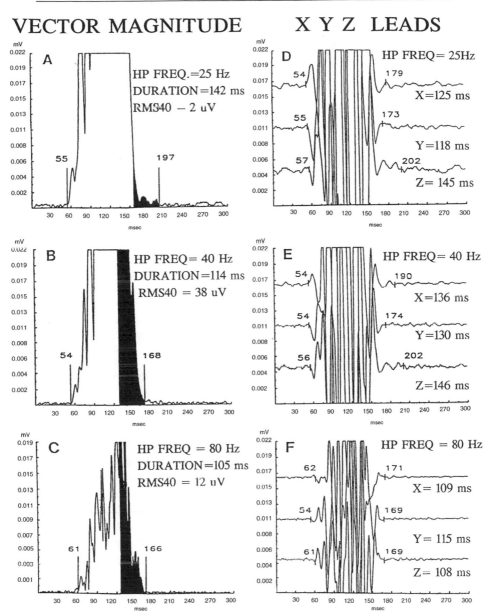

Figure 5.1. Demonstration of the effects of the high-pass cutoff frequency on the individual XYZ leads and the resulting filtered vector magnitude. Panels **A** and **D** were filtered at 25 Hz, panels **B** and **E** were filtered at 40 Hz, and panels **C** and **F** were filtered at 80 Hz.

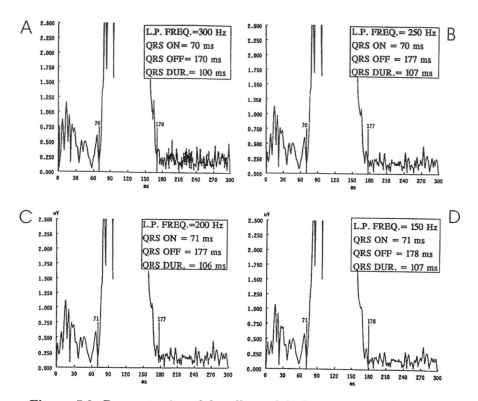

Figure 5.2. Demonstration of the effects of the low-pass cutoff frequency on the filtered vector magnitude. Panels **A–H** were filtered at 300 Hz, 250 Hz, 200 Hz, 150 Hz, 100 Hz, 75 Hz, 50 Hz, and 25 Hz, respectively. (Reprinted with permission of Futura Publishing Company.[11])

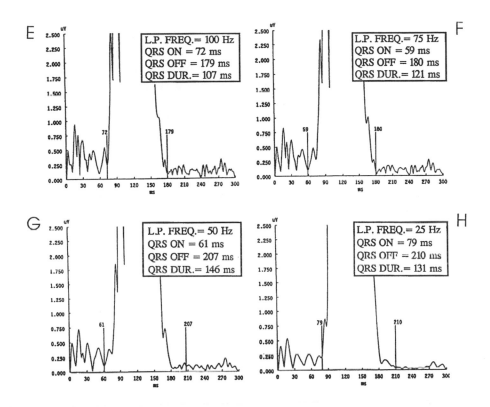

low-frequency response, such as analog tape-based Holter recorders, are very prone to analysis errors.

Automatic Measurement Algorithms

SAECG devices use computer software to identify the QRS_{offset} and QRS_{onset} points. As discussed in Chapter 4, all of the standard late potential parameters rely particularly on the QRS_{offset} point. The precision with which both points are chosen can greatly affect the numerical values of the late potential parameters. Knowing how these points are determined will enable the reader to judge their validity and develop the skill for identifying errors due to artifacts.

In general, the methods used to identify the QRS_{offset} and QRS_{onset} points are based on measuring an average value in two adjacent windows of the filtered vector magnitude. Figure 5.3 shows a filtered vector magnitude recording and on the right side are two data windows labeled A and B. The average value of the signal is calculated in both windows along with the standard deviation of window B. The two averages are compared and when the difference between them exceeds three times the value of the standard deviation of

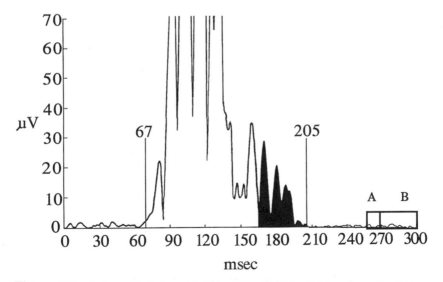

Figure 5.3. Automatic determination of the QRS_{offset} is based on calculating the average voltage in two adjacent regions of the filtered vector magnitude, labeled A and B. These windows "slide" toward the end of the QRS, and when the average value of A exceeds the average value of B by three standard deviations, then the QRS_{offset} is determined.

window B, then the QRS_{offset} is defined at that point. If this is not the case then both windows are advanced one point closer to the QRS complex and the process is repeated. In a similar fashion the QRS_{onset} is determined but with shorter duration windows and a larger number of standard deviation differences, e.g., five times.

Of particular note is the fact that the QRS_{onset} is calculated on the *unfiltered* vector magnitude. The reason for this is demonstrated in Figure 5.4. Panel A shows the unfiltered XYZ leads and panel B is the unfiltered vector magnitude derived from these leads. Panel C is the usual filtered vector magnitude. Two vertical lines are drawn through the three panels. The left-most line is where the automatic algorithm chose the QRS_{onset} using the filtered vector magnitude (panel C) and the right-most line is where the automatic algorithm chose the QRS_{onset} using the unfiltered vector magnitude (panel B). Note that there is a 10-msec difference between these two points. A systematic study comparing these two methods[11] showed at least a 10-msec difference in 90 of 100 patients studied. The reason for this is that the early ventricular signal in the high-resolution filtered vector magnitude is most likely His-Purkinje activity. The His-Purkinje signals were the primary focus of the initial application of the SAECG. Historically, measures of the onset of ventricular activation begin with myocardial muscle activation and do not include signals from the His-Purkinje system.

The QRS_{offset} point, when determined with either the automatic algorithms or with visual inspection, does not necessarily define the end of ventricular depolarization. After all of the processing steps, such as signal averaging and high-pass filtering, it is still possible that ventricular depolarization signals that are extremely small may still be undetectable. Such small late potential signals have been studied[12] but without a means of verification. Several human and canine studies have attempted to correlate direct recording electrograms with the body surface recordings.[13-15] There is ample evidence that the filtered vector magnitude will not detect the longest duration late potentials and that individual lead analysis will significantly improve upon the vector magnitude for recording the full extent of late potential activity.

The Effects of Noise on Late Potential Measurements

The primary reason to perform signal averaging is to reduce the amount of noise in a high-resolution recording. However, there will

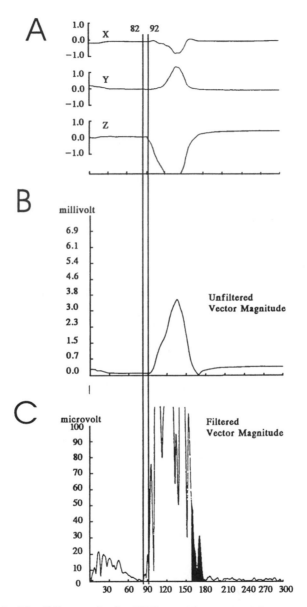

Figure 5.4. The difference in the QRS$_{onset}$ as determined from the unfiltered vector magnitude and the filtered vector magnitude using an automatic algorithm approach similar to the process shown in Figure 5.3. In this case the filtered vector magnitude QRS$_{onset}$ was 10 msec earlier than in the unfiltered vector magnitude. (Reprinted with permission of the Journal of Electrocardiology.[12])

always be some level of residual noise remaining due to fundamental limitations and the practicality of the recording environment. There have been studies that examine the role of this residual noise and the clinical performance of the SAECG.[16,17] Quantifying noise is not uniformly performed in the commercial systems; however, most use some measure of noise to provide a uniform endpoint for the SAECG. An interesting example of the use of the noise function described in the previous chapter is shown in Figure 5.5. On the left side are two filtered vector magnitude recordings from the same patient but at two different sampling rates. The time window in panel A was 300 msec and it appeared that the entire post-QRS period was contaminated with a large amount of noise (estimated average of 5.0 μV) since there was no return to the noise baseline apparent in the recording. Panel B shows the noise function for the signal in panel A. Note the natural progression to decreasing noise to a final value of 0.3 μV when about 217 beats were averaged. This low level and continual reduction in noise indicates a valid signal-averaged recording. Panel C is from the same patient with the time window increases to 600 msec. The corresponding noise function is in panel D. This noise function behaves similarly to the one in panel B, also implying a valid signal-averaged recording. It is apparent in panel C that the late potential signal eventually decreases in amplitude to a base noise level and that the post-QRS noise in panel A was indeed a late potential signal.

The accuracy of the QRS_{onset} and QRS_{offset} points is directly related to the amount of residual noise in the signal-averaged waveforms. As could be deduced from the description of the automatic algorithms, the greater the noise, the more difficult the task of identifying the QRS endpoints. Figure 5.6 shows an example of two filtered vector magnitude recordings from the same patient. Panel A was the result of averaging 200 beats and panel B represents an average of 600 beats. Theoretically, a 600-beat average would result in noise levels about 50% lower than a 200-beat average. This can be subjectively viewed in the post-QRS period of both panels. The automatic algorithm for choosing the QRSd shows a 4-msec difference between the two averages: 159 msec in panel A versus 163 msec in panel B. This is an error of about 2.5%, presuming that the lower noise average is the more accurate measurement of QRSd. There is a 1-msec difference in choosing the QRS_{onset} compared to a 5-msec difference in identifying the QRS_{offset}. The more remarkable difference occurs in the RMS40 measurement. The error is on the order of 100%; from

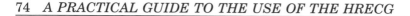

VECTOR MAGNITUDE   NOISE FUNCTION

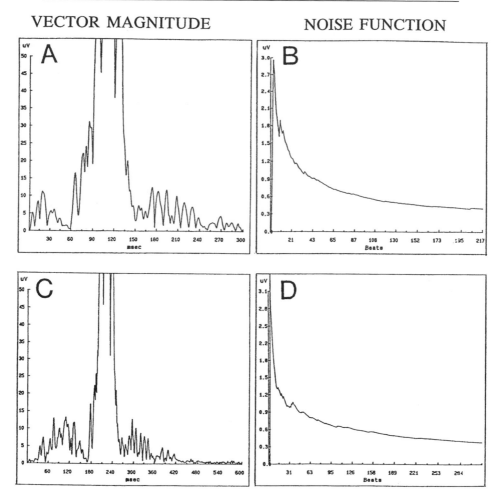

Figure 5.5. Apparent high levels of noise (estimated average of about 5.0 μV) in the post-QRS region of the filtered vector magnitude (panel **A**) but with a decreasing noise function measurement to about 0.3 μV. Slowing the sampling rate increases the time window from 300 msec to 600 msec (panel **C**), and the end of the late potential region is more apparent. The noise function measurement in panel **D** shows an almost identical character as the one in panel **B**.

14.29 μV to 27.57 μV. This large difference was alluded to in Chapter 4 where the RMS40 measurement was discussed in more detail.

The sensitivity of the late potential measurements to residual noise is the primary reason that signal-averaging software will calculate noise levels during the averaging process. This use of noise

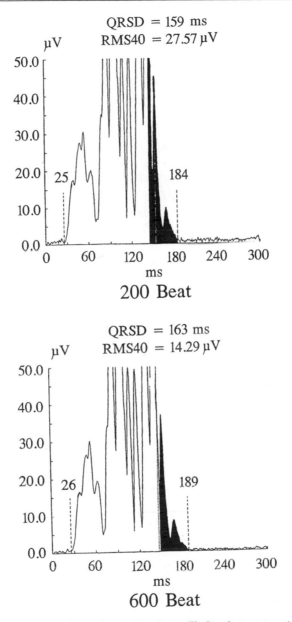

Figure 5.6. Residual noise after averaging will alter late potential measurements when comparing a 200-beat average (**top**) with a 600-beat (**bottom**). The QRSd increases by only a few percent, but the RMS40 decreases by almost 50%.

estimation has greatly improved the reproducibility and standardization of the SAECG.

Bundle Branch Block and Intraventricular Conduction Defects

From the earliest use of the SAECG, it was recognized that the inclusion of patients with a bundle branch block (BBB) had to be considered separately from those without BBB. The fundamental problem is that the wide QRS of BBB is due to the late activation of normal myocardium. On the SAECG, it is impossible to distinguish these apparent late potentials from those originating from the scarred infarcted regions. Figure 5.7 from Buckingham et al.[18] shows four filtered vector magnitude recordings. Panel A is from a normal patient without VT; panel B is from a patient with normal fascicular activation of the ventricles and with VT; panels C and D are from patients with left BBB without VT (panel C) and with VT (panel D). The point of this figure is to show qualitatively that there are no identifiable differences among patients with BBB block with and without VT. For this reason, the use of time domain methods cannot be used for late potential quantification in patients with BBB.

Antiarrhythmic Drugs and Late Potentials

Another factor that can influence the QRS duration and late potential characteristics is the presence of an antiarrhythmic drug. Those drugs that block sodium channels (so-called class I drugs) will slow conduction and result in a longer duration QRS complex. Such drugs will also slow conduction in regions of late potential sources and will then add further to the increased duration of the QRS as measured in the SAECG. Several studies have examined the role of such drugs on the SAECG and have demonstrated that there may be a more pronounced suppression of conduction within the late potential substrate than in the normal ventricular muscle.[19-21] This differential effect would result in a proportionately longer late potential signal than the main body of the QRS complex. Figure 5.8 shows an example of the effects of propafenone on the standard QRSd, the rate of an induced VT, and the filtered vector magnitude of the SAECG in a patient before (top panel) and after (bottom panel) drug administration. The standard ECG showed a change in the QRS of 10 msec and the tachycardia cycle length was lengthened from 265

BUNDLE BRANCH BLOCK

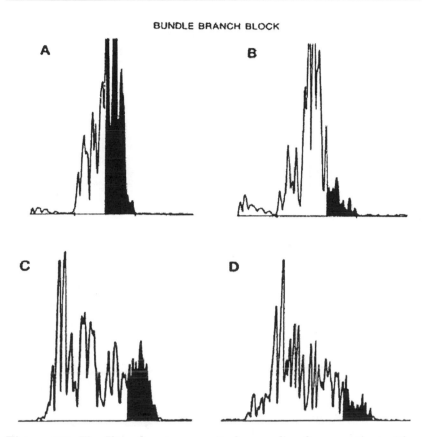

Figure 5.7. The filtered vector magnitude recording from a patient with a normally conducted QRS and no VT is shown in panel **A**. Panel **B** is from a patient with a normally conducted QRS, but with VT. Panels **C** and **D** are from patients with left BBB without VT (panel **C**) and with ventricular tachycardia (panel **D**). (Reprinted with permission of the American Journal of Cardiology.[18])

msec to 380 msec. The QRSd increased from 151 msec to 177 msec. Of this overall change of 26 msec, the authors make the case that 20 msec of this change was in the late potentials versus only 6 msec in the main body of the QRS complex.

Artifacts and Quality Control

Signal averaging is a statistical process. Several assumptions are made about the signal of interest and the underlying noise. The signal is assumed to be repeatable in every beat that is included

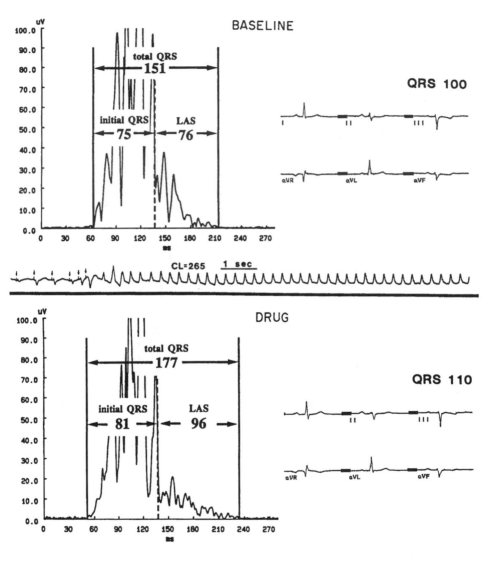

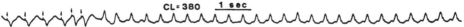

Figure 5.8. The effects of propafenone on the QRS complex, VT cycle length, and the SAECG. The top panel is from a patient prior to drug administration and the bottom panel is after drug administration. (Reprinted with permission of the American College of Cardiology.[19])

in the average. Also, the noise and the signal are assumed to be independent from each other and the noise is assumed to be random. In practice, these assumptions are usually true, but there are situations in which these assumptions are false and the result would be an invalid average. For example, the detection, classification, and alignment of each beat are all performed in software, and depending on the particular implementation, the user will have a varying degree of observation or control of these parts of the system. An example of how a false positive result can occur is in the case of including a premature ventricular beat in the average or a misalignment of a normal beat due to an artifact. This type of error is simulated in the Figure 5.9. Panel A is the filtered vector magnitude from a 25-year-old normal male subject. Panels B-D were obtained with the same

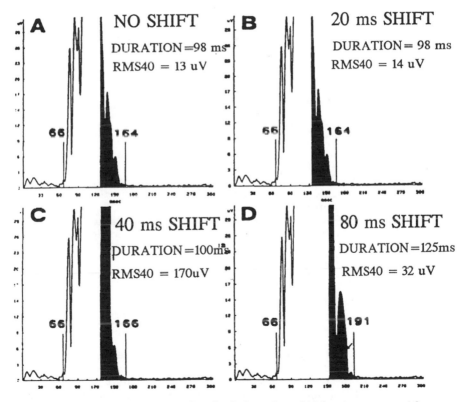

Figure 5.9. Misalignment of a single beat in a 200-beat average with an alignment shift of 20 msec, 40 msec, and 80 msec shown in panels **B**, **C**, and **D**, respectively. (Reprinted with permission of the Journal of Electrocardiology.[12])

set of data except that one beat was shifted in time by 20 msec, 40 msec, or 80 msec, respectively. There are about 200 beats in the original average and the error rate for proper beat detection is 0.5%. Note that the QRSd in panel D is 125 msec and would indicate an abnormal value for this SAECG.

It is important understand that an average could be invalid due to a technical failure, but repeating the average allows the reader to examine the reproducibility of the late potentials. It is usually best to directly visualize the waveform morphologies and not just the derived late potential parameters.

References

1. Okin PM, Stein KM, Lippman N, Lerman BB, Kligfield P. Performance of the signal-averaged electrocardiogram: Relation to baseline QRS duration. Am Heart J 129(5):932-940, 1995.
2. Macfarlane PW, Chen CY, Chiang BN. Comparison of the ECG in apparently healthy Chinese and Caucasians. Computers in Cardiology, IEEE Computer Society Press, 1988, pp 143-146.
3. Lander P, Berbari EJ, Rajagopalan CV, Vatterott P, Lazzara R. Critical analysis of the signal-averaged electrocardiogram: Improved identification of late potentials. Circulation 87:105-117, 1993.
4. Yang TF, Macfarlane PW. New sex dependent normal limits of the signal averaged electrocardiogram. Br Heart J 72:197-200, 1994.
5. Macfarlane PW, Veitch Lawrie TD (eds). Comprehensive Electrocardiology: Theory and Practice in Health and Disease, Volumes 1-3, Pergamon Press, England, 1989.
6. Hayabuchi Y, Matsuoka S, Kubo M, Akita H, Kuroda Y. Age-related criteria for signal-averaged electrocardiographic late potentials in children. Pediatr Cardiol 15:107-111, 1994.
7. Savard P, Rouleau JL, Ferguson J, et al. Risk stratification after myocardial infarction using signal-averaged electrocardiographic criteria adjusted for sex, age, and myocardial infarction location. Circulation 96:202-213, 1997.
8. Simson MB. Use of signals in the terminal QRS complex to identify patients with ventricular tachycardia after myocardial infarction. Circulation 64:235, 1981.
9. Gomes JA, Winters SL, Stewart D, Targonski A, Barreca P. Optimal bandpass filters for time-domain analysis of the signal-averaged electrocardiogram. Am J Cardiol 60:1290-1298, 1987.
10. Bragg-Remschel DA, Anderson CM, Winkle RA. Frequency response characteristics of ambulatory ECG monitoring systems and their implications for ST segment analysis. Am Heart J 103:20-31, 1982.
11. Berbari EJ, Rajagopalan CV, Lander P, Lazzara R. Changes in late potential measurements as a function of decreasing bandwidth. J Cardiovasc Electrophysiol 2:503-508, 1991.
12. Berbari EJ, Lander P, Scherlag BJ. Verification of the high resolution electrocardiogram. J Electrocardiol 22(Suppl):1-6, 1989.

13. Simson MB, Euler D, Michelson EL, Falcone RA, Spear JF, Moore EN. Detection of delayed ventricular activation on the body surface in dogs. Am J Physiol 241:H363-H368, 1981.
14. Simson MB, Untereker WJ, Spielman ST, et al. Relation between late potentials on the body surface and directly recorded fragmented electrograms in patients with ventricular tachycardia. Am J Cardiol 51:105-112, 1983.
15. Berbari EJ, Lander P, Geselowitz DB, Scherlag BJ, Lazzara R. Identifying the end of ventricular activation: Body surface late potentials versus electrogram measurements in a canine infarction model. J Cardiovasc Electrophysiol 5(1):28-40, 1994.
16. Vatterott PJ, Hammill SC, Berbari EJ, et al. The effect of residual noise on the reproducibility of the signal averaged ECG. J Electrocardiol 20 (Suppl): 102, 1987.
17. Steinberg JS, Bigger JT. Importance of the endpoint of noise reduction in analysis of the signal-averaged electrocardiogram. Am J Cardiol 63:556-560, 1989.
18. Buckingham TA, Thessen CC, Steven LL, Redd RM, Kennedy HL. Effect of conduction defects on the signal-averaged electrocardiographic determination of late potentials. Am J Cardiol 61:1265-1271, 1988.
19. Freedman RA, Steinberg JS. Selective prolongation of QRS late potentials by sodium channel blocking antiarrhythmic drugs: Relation to slowing ventricular tachycardia. J Am Coll Cardiol 17:1017-1025, 1991.
20. Freedman RA, Karagounis LA, Steinberg JS. Effects of sotalol on the signal-averaged electrocardiogram in patients with sustained ventricular tachycardia: Relation to suppression of inducibility and changes in tachycardia cycle length. J Am Coll Cardiol 20:1213-1219, 1992.
21. Greenspon AJ, Kidwell GA, DeCaro M, Hessen S. The effects of type I antiarrhythmic drugs on the signal-averaged electrocardiogram in patients with malignant ventricular arrhythmias. PACE 15:1445-1453, 1992.

6

The Signal-Averaged Electrocardiogram in Clinical Practice

Establishing the Clinical Utility of the Signal-Averaged Electrocardiogram

The gold standard by which a clinical test should be judged is the accurate prediction of an appropriate, well-defined endpoint in a large, unselected patient population followed prospectively for a suitable duration of time. Design and performance of such an investigation is by definition a major undertaking. It has been common to "break ground" with a new clinical test by describing its performance using retrospective data or referred "post-event" patient samples. Although the data derived from such studies are not always confirmed in prospective, clinical investigations, the SAECG had its clinical birth in this manner. In certain clinical contexts, no other data exist and therefore the clinician must extrapolate imperfect observations to the real world of clinical practice.

Introduction of the Signal-Averaged Electrocardiogram to Clinical Practice

In 1981, Dr. Michael Simson[1] published the initial experience with the SAECG used to identify patients with ventricular tachycardia (VT). The technique for recording and analysis described in this article laid much of the foundation for the clinical application of SAECG as a research tool and noninvasive test in clinical practice.

Surface leads were constructed as a three-polar lead configuration, X, Y, and Z. The ECG signal was amplified and A to D converted at 1000 samples/sec. Template recognition was used for rejection of ectopic or excessively noisy beats. Each averaged lead was filtered with a bidirectional digital filter to limit nonlinear phase shifts at the end of the QRS complex. The high-pass filter frequency was 25 Hz and the low-pass filter frequency was 250 Hz. The three leads were combined into a vector magnitude. The onset and offset of the filtered QRS complex were defined as the segments that exceeded the mean plus three standard deviations of the noise sample. The total duration of filtered QRS was measured. In addition, the RMS voltage was calculated in the terminal 40 msec of the QRS, an interval that represented the period of a 25-Hz waveform.

The study group included 39 patients with remote myocardial infarction (MI) who had recurrent episodes of spontaneous sustained VT and inducible VT at electrophysiological study (EPS). This group was contrasted with a select group of 27 patients, many with recent MI, who had no spontaneous ventricular ectopy on 24-hour ambulatory ECGs and who had no episodes of sustained VT. Simson[1] observed that patients without VT had a rapid decline of high-frequency energy at the end of the QRS, whereas the VT patients had lower high-frequency voltage but the voltage declined more gradually and generally outlasted the QRS duration (QRSd) of control patients, i.e., a late potential. The terminal signals were not discrete but were continuous with the main portion of the QRS. In fact, the QRSd of the filtered complex was about 45 msec longer and the terminal voltage was one fifth lower in patients with VT in contrast to the control patients. The total QRS voltage did not differ greatly between groups. An SAECG QRSd exceeding 120 msec and a voltage in the last 40 msec of the QRS below 25 mV effectively discriminated the two groups. Although notching of the late portion of the unfiltered QRS complex was frequently observed in the VT patients, it was also common in the patients after MI who had no VT.

The study elegantly demonstrated the feasibility of signal-averaged recording and interpretation in patients with coronary heart disease, the potential to distinguish MI associated with VT from MI without VT, and the presumed noninvasive correlate of slow conduction required for reentry.

A large examination of the relationship of late potentials and the presence of coronary artery disease and ventricular wall motion abnormality was conducted by Breithardt et al. in 1982.[2] The study was the first clinical one that looked at normal subjects and found that visually defined late potentials were not detected in the absence of structural heart disease. The presence of late potentials and their duration were significantly greater in patients who had a history of sustained ventricular tachyarrhythmias. For example, late potentials had a duration of 51 msec when there was a previous history of VT or ventricular fibrillation (VF) compared to only 31 msec in patients with no such history. Late potentials were identified in 71% of patients when there was a history of sustained ventricular arrhythmia but in only 28% when there was not. One of the most important findings in this analysis was that the presence of late potentials was strongly related to the presence of left ventricular dysfunction. When left ventricular function was normal, only 9% had late potentials and these were all of short duration. The greater the severity of left ventricular dysfunction, the more frequently were late potentials detected. Because this study was a nonprospective investigation, it was unclear whether the false positive findings in patients with ventricular wall motion abnormality would be a major impediment to the use of the SAECG as a clinical tool for the prediction of VT. In fact, in subsequent prospective analysis,[3,4] ventricular function was found to be at most only weakly related to the presence of SAECG abnormalities or late potentials. The discrepancy in these findings probably results from the referred population studied by Breithardt et al.[2] compared to consecutively enrolled patients following acute MI in the prospective investigations.

The finding of longer duration late potentials in patients with sustained VTs may have physiological significance. If greater degrees of conduction delay are present in sinus rhythm, it may be that less "stress" may be required for conduction to further prolong and to complete a reentrant circuit. In fact, the number of repetitive ventricular responses to programmed electrical stimulation has been correlated to the duration of late potentials.[5] It may also be observed that VT will be slower if the SAECG has late potentials of greater duration,[5,6] which may indicate a greater volume of slow conducting tissue participating in the tachycardia circuit. However, the bulk of the evidence suggests that late potentials indicate only indirectly the presence of slow conducting tissue and do not necessarily indicate the tissue that will participate in the subsequent reentrant circuit and thus may not be highly accurate in predicting the ease of inducibility, the tachycardia cycle length, the frequency of arrhythmia occurrence, and other similarly related characteristics.

Not surprisingly, there is no correlation between the local refractory period recorded in the right ventricle at EPS and SAECG indices.[7] The SAECG is a measure of the depolarization process and ventricular conduction and typically indicates ventricular activation delay in the left ventricle, so that the lack of correlation between refractoriness and SAECG would be expected.

There are clearly differences in the strength of the association of the SAECG and the type of clinical arrhythmia or the arrhythmia induced at EPS. It has previously been shown that the SAECG has the strongest relationship with clinical and induced sustained monomorphic VT, but the relationship is less strong when the arrhythmia is either nonsustained VT or is VF. For example, longer filtered QRSds were present in patients with inducible sustained monomorphic VT, whereas patients with inducible sustained polymorphic VT or VF and patients with inducible nonsustained VT had QRSds approximately 10 msec shorter; however, both groups had much longer filtered QRSds than patients who had noninducible arrhythmias at EPS.[7]

Concerns have been raised that patients who experience more rapid VTs including VF may have lesser degrees of conduction delay and less abnormality on the SAECG. Previous studies have suggested that the longer the duration of the late potential, the longer the VT cycle length.[5,6] Freedman et al.[8] compared the SAECG findings in 24 patients who had experienced at least one episode of VF and 27 patients who had experienced at least one episode of spontaneous sustained VT. Although important SAECG abnormalities were detected between these groups of patients, there were also important clinical characteristics that differed between the groups. Patients with VT were younger, less often male, and more often had nonischemic heart disease. There was also a trend for these patients to have better preserved left ventricular function. As expected at EPS, patients with VF generally did not have inducible sustained VT, whereas patients with clinical VT often did. In regard to the SAECG, patients with clinical VT had lower values of terminal voltage. In fact, patients with VF more closely resembled normal patients in the distribution of terminal voltage values. Finally, lower values of terminal voltage (RMS40) were found in those with inducible sustained VTs compared with those who had no arrhythmia or nonsustained arrhythmias induced regardless of clinical presentation. Overall, the study identified an abnormal terminal voltage value in only 21% of patients with VF. These SAECG findings are in accord with differences in clinical characteristics, inducible ventricular arrhythmia and endocardial or epicardial recordings from the surface of the heart. It is entirely possible that the greater the degree of slow conduction present, the more likely the patients will have VT both in the EP laboratory and as a clinical event. Experimental work in animal preparations also suggest that inducible VF is associated with less conduction delay and therefore the arrhythmogenic substrate that can sustain VT.[9,10] Presumably less conduction slowing may lead to more rapid ventricular arrhythmias and a greater propensity to degeneration to VF. However, these findings highlight one of the limitations in SAECG recording: lower sensitivity to predict the most malignant of VTs and more accurate prediction of those sustained arrhythmias that would be less likely fatal.

Prospective Investigation: Spontaneous Arrhythmic Events

Time Course of Signal-Averaged Electrocardiogram Abnormality Early after Acute Myocardial Infarction and Relationship to Early Ventricular Arrhythmias

Experimental work has shown that delayed, fractionated electrical activity can be recorded from the ischemic zone within minutes of coronary artery occlusion in dog models.[11] Because the chronic substrate for late ventricular arrhythmias is fibrosis and the resultant derangement of myocardial cellular architecture[12] is not present for at least several days after MI, early conduction abnormalities likely result from abnormal cellular electrical function. Thus, changes recorded early after MI do not reflect the same pathophysiology as recording days or weeks later. At best, they can indicate a predisposition to development of later structural alterations that are responsible for the electrophysiological milieu of VT. Myocardial cellular uncoupling[13] that is present in the days after MI may evolve into the fibrosis of a healed MI. Both can cause conduction delay. Early recordings will also be influenced by abnormalities resulting from remote myocardial damage, and without prior tracings for comparison, distinction between new and old SAECG irregularities is not possible.

Serial SAECGs were recorded in 50 patients during the first 10 days of hospitalization after acute MI by McGuire et al.[14] There was a progressive increase in the prevalence of patients with abnormal SAECG recordings, from 32% during the first 24 hours to 52% on days 7-10. The development of a late potential on any recording during the hospital stay was not related to any measured clinical variable, especially size of MI. Patients who developed sustained ventricular arrhythmia during the in-hospital phase of recovery from

MI were more likely to have abnormal SAECG parameters; however, the SAECG was recorded after the event in many patients. In contrast, Kertes et al.[15] found a low prevalence of late potentials early after MI that declined further during hospitalization, and that did not correlate with early onset VF. Both studies [14,15] were relatively small, and the presence of VT in some patients in the McGuire study rather than solely VF in the Kertes[15] study may account for the differences in results. Gomes et al.[16] also noted no correlation between clinical features and SAECG findings when recorded approximately 3 days after MI.

In a larger study of 281 patients performed by Hong et al.,[17] the occurrence of VT/VF during the first 48 hours of hospitalization was strongly associated with an abnormal SAECG reading on day 5. Interestingly, the unfiltered QRS (comparable to that obtained from the standard ECG) did not differ between patients with and without ventricular arrhythmia. Larger infarcts were associated with early ventricular arrhythmia, but the presence of late potentials retained an independent association. Interestingly, the acute phase ventricular arrhythmias after coronary occlusion may be due to enhanced automaticity[18] and thus independent of conduction delay that the SAECG is designed to detect.

In aggregate, these studies show an association between SAECG abnormality and early ventricular arrhythmia, primarily VF. However, the clinical utility of these observations is limited. There is no purpose in recording the SAECG after acute VT/VF has occurred because it develops in a relatively short circumscribed time frame of 24-48 hours, and often before hospitalization. In addition, the technical difficulties of very early recording (e.g., on admission) or in the coronary care unit need to be emphasized.

Predischarge Risk Stratification after Acute Myocardial Infarction: Use of the Signal-Averaged Electrocardiogram and Other Noninvasive and Invasive Variables

The Signal-Averaged Electrocardiogram as a Tool for Risk Prediction

After MI, the necrotic tissue is replaced by fibrous tissue, resulting in scar formation. This healing process may disrupt the normal architecture of human myocardium and may have devastating consequences on the passage of electrical current (see Chapter 2). In its aftermath, the healed MI perpetuates a permanent risk for lethal ventricular arrhythmias by a complex and not fully understood interaction of fixed electrical abnormality and transient factors (e.g., ischemia, alterations in autonomic balance, ventricular ectopy, ventricular filling pressures, etc.).

In the aftermath of MI, patients remain at risk for life-threatening complications. About half of the deaths that occur in the population of patients with healed MI occur rapidly and without warning. This devastating scenario is generally referred to as sudden cardiac death. Electrocardiographic recordings during these events support the premise that these events are arrhythmic, and in the vast majority of cases are due to ventricular tachyarrhythmias, VT, and VF. Although some, perhaps many, of sudden cardiac deaths may occur on the basis of coronary ischemia, many such patients have neither clinical nor pathological evidence of ischemia. These patients presumably have a fixed permanent risk of VT and VF due to the pathology of MI, although many factors may influence the timing, frequency, and severity of arrhythmia development.

The greatest risk of death after MI is in the weeks and months following hospital discharge. Thereafter (after approximately 6-12 months), the risk diminishes and remains constant unless a new cardiac event supervenes. This early high risk places a specific burden on risk stratification efforts. Risk prediction must be performed early enough to identify those in the high attrition group and to permit effective intervention, if appropriate, for these patients.

There have been multiple studies that have prospectively identified patients after MI, recorded the SAECG, and then followed the patients for the development of spontaneous sustained ventricular arrhythmias or sudden cardiac (and presumed arrhythmic) death. The studies differ somewhat in enrollment criteria and often in SAECG methodology, but have been remarkably uniform in their conclusions.

In 1983, Breithardt et al.[19] published the first study that recognized the prognostic importance of the SAECG. Recruited from several hospitals between 7 and 109 days after acute MI, 160 patients were enrolled. The SAECG was recorded as four bipolar precordial leads and then filtered at 100-300 Hz with a single pole analog filter. Late potentials were visually identified from the high-gain signal-averaged recordings as low-amplitude activity at the end of the QRS. Although there was no objective definition to the late potential, its duration was estimated from the onset of low-amplitude activity to the end of the signal.

A relatively high proportion of patients met the criteria for late potentials (51%), but late potentials of >20 msec were observed in only 30%. Approximately twice as many patients with posterior MI had late potentials compared to the patients with anterior MI. There was a trend for patients with larger infarcts (as assessed enzymatically) to have longer late potentials. There was, however, no relationship between late potential presence or duration and the presence of ventricular ectopy on ECG monitoring.

Follow-up in this study was relatively brief, only 7.5 months. Although there was a trend for patients who experienced sudden death, symptomatic VT, or cardiac death to have late potentials more commonly, the association was not statistically significant. Similarly, the late potentials were longer in patients who experienced arrhythmic endpoints than in those who did not, but they were of insufficient magnitude to reach statistical significance. When patients were grouped by the absence of a late potential or the presence of a short duration late potential (<20 msec), there was a lower incidence of sustained VT (0%) and sudden death (3.8%) than in their counterparts with prolonged late potentials (p<0.01). Those patients with the longest late potentials (>40 msec) had a sudden death rate of 11% and a VT rate of 17% in short-term follow-up. Figure 6.1 is a bar graph summarizing these relationships. Arrhythmic events were more common in patients with anterior MI, although the SAECG was more commonly abnormal in posterior MI.

This first prospective study showed that late potentials were commonly detected after MI, were related to the site of MI, and could possibly predict the first occurrence of VT or VF. However, the study was relatively small with brief follow-up and primitive technology, so that further investigation was warranted.

A few years later, several publications appeared in the cardiology literature, which furthered the investigation of Breithardt et al.[19] These studies began to utilize a quantitative approach to SAECG analysis, based to a large extent on the work of Simson.[1] Quantitative analysis lends itself to greater precision, can minimize investigator bias, and facilitates comparisons between and among investigative and clinical centers. The quantitative details used from study to study differed slightly and partially account for differences in the incidence of SAECG abnormalities and to a lesser extent clinical endpoints.

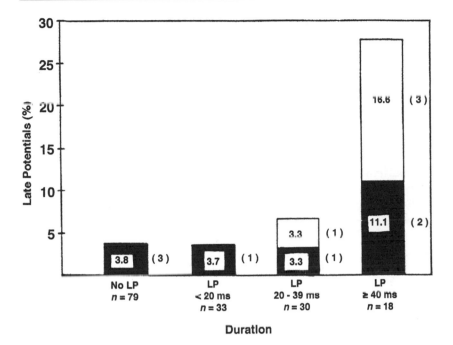

Figure 6.1. In a post-MI prospective study, relationship of the presence of duration and late potentials to subsequent ventricular (white area) and sudden death (black area). LP = late potential. (Reprinted with permission from European Heart Journal; Breithardt et al.[19])

In a study of 165 patients, Kuchar et al.[20] performed SAECG as well as Holter ECG and left ventricular ejection fraction (LVEF) before hospital discharge. Patients were followed for at least 6 months.

The SAECG revealed an abnormality in 41% of patients, a low terminal amplitude primarily and a prolonged filtered QRS less often. There was evidence that patients with an abnormal SAECG tracing had larger infarcts; these patients had higher peak MB fraction of creatine kinase and lower LVEF. As in the Breithardt study,[19] an inferior site of MI was more heavily represented in the group with abnormal SAECG results.

Kuchar et al.[20] also examined the evolution of the SAECG in the first year post-MI. Overall, the filtered QRSd remained the same during serial assessment. Although QRSd was stable, the voltage in the terminal 40 msec of the QRS increased from hospital discharge until 6 weeks but thereafter remained stable. Of the sizable group of patients who had an abnormal SAECG at hospital discharge, there was a progressive pattern of normalization over time; at 1 year, 30% had normalized. Normalization was due principally to an increase in the terminal QRS voltage and not due to a change in QRSd[20]; this observation raises the question of whether the changes were on a technical basis rather than a genuine evolution of pathophysiological substrate.

Cardiac events classified as ventricular arrhythmias were observed in 8% of the study cohort, and were much more common in the patients whose SAECGs were abnormal. Survival without an arrhythmic event to 1 year was 99% in the patients with normal SAECGs but only 83% in the group with abnormal SAECGs, a difference that was highly statistically significant. Although the SAECG had good sensitivity and moderate specificity, the positive predictive accuracy was fairly low.

The finding of a low positive predictive value is common in the SAECG literature, but this observation is not unlike values seen for other commonly performed noninvasive tests post-MI. For example, for an LVEF of <40% and for an abnormal Holter reading, the positive predictive values were 23% and 17%, respectively, in the Kuchar study.[20]

Even though the risk of an arrhythmic event was vastly higher for the patients with abnormal SAECGs, the great majority of this subset did not experience an event in follow-up. To place these findings in context, one must bear in mind that the predictive value in prospective studies is not only dependent on the intrinsic value of the specific test, but also on the event rate in the population studied, which in turn depends on the characteristics of the patients and the duration of follow-up. Most events, however, tend to cluster in the first 3 to 6 months after MI.

Most prospective studies of SAECG or other noninvasive tests perform the test in question prior to hospital discharge. The rationale of this timing is both practical and scientific. Enrollment of study patients after MI is facilitated when they are inpatients. Furthermore, the first few months after MI have the highest event rate. Although the evolution of the pathological substrate after MI is probably incomplete at this stage, it is relatively mature and largely reflective of the final pathological state. Thus, the most common time of SAECG recording was around days 10–14 post-MI in the clinical trials; clinical implications of SAECG use are based on this premise.

In a large prospective study of patients who had survived an uncomplicated MI, Denniss et al.[21] examined the prognostic value of programmed ventricular stimulation and "delayed potentials" from the SAECG. Delayed potentials were defined by visual interpretation of a high-gain unfiltered three-lead ECG when the QRSd exceeded 140 msec. Over 300 patients were enrolled and patients with bundle branch block (BBB) were excluded.

The SAECG revealed delayed potentials in 26% of patients and their presence was associated with evidence of large acute MI and its aftermath (increased maximum CK level, higher Norris index, and longer His-Purkinje conduction time). An important and unique observation was the correlation of VT inducibility by programmed stimulation and the presence of delayed potentials (see below). Patients who exhibited delayed potentials were no more likely to have provocable ischemia on treadmill testing or to have more extensive coronary artery disease. Left ventricular dysfunction was greater, however, in the group with delayed potentials. Thus, the SAECG was more likely to be abnormal when there was more extensive myocardial damage assessed by a variety of indices, but not necessarily when the ischemic risk was more burdensome. Interestingly, delayed ventricular activation as detected by the SAECG was not associated with delayed repolarization (QT and QTc) as measured on the ECG.

During follow-up, only a minority of patients were treated with chronic beta-blocker therapy, which may in part account for the relatively high event rate. In addition, a component of the study cohort were participants in a trial of antiarrhythmic drug therapy; patients with delayed potentials were more than twice as likely to have received antiarrhythmic drugs in follow-up. With these qualifications in mind, the occurrence of fatal or nonfatal cardiac events was far more likely when the SAECG was abnormal. For example, because the event rate was high, this study was the first to demonstrate a significant advantage in overall survival in the patients with normal SAECG results.[20] This difference was further magnified when the combined endpoint of instantaneous death and sustained ventricular arrhythmias was analyzed. Patients without delayed potentials had an event rate of only 2% at 1 year and 4% at 2 years, compared with event rates of 15% and 21% at 1 and 2 years, respectively, when delayed potentials were detected. This striking contrast in outcome was highly statistically significant; the presence of delayed potentials was associated with a sixfold increase in risk of fatal and nonfatal ventricular arrhythmias and fourfold increase in risk of cardiac death.

Using the Signal-Averaged Electrocardiogram in Combination with Other Noninvasive Test Results to Predict Serious Ventricular Arrhythmias after Myocardial Infarction

In the early 1980s, it became firmly established that the LVEF and the frequency and complexity of ventricular arrhythmia on Holter ECG could predict the development of sustained ventricular arrhythmias after acute MI.[22] A complete discussion of these findings is beyond the scope of this presentation, but several critical findings will be described. Mortality is strongly related to the radionuclide ejection fraction measured in the convalescent phase of acute MI.[22] In one large study, the 2-year mortality rate was only 6% if the LVEF was > 40%, which was in striking contrast to the 50% mortality rate if the LVEF was < 20%.[22] LVEF was an independent predictor and imparted an eightfold increase in risk of mortality when the LVEF was <40%. Holter-detected ventricular arrhythmia also predicted risk. When the frequency of ventricular premature beats was at least 10 per hour, the mortality rate was increased approximately threefold. The presence of repetitive forms (couplets and nonsustained VT) also predicted mortality, and the increment in risk was independent of the frequency of ventricular premature beats. Finally, the mortality risk was independently increased by the presence of left ventricular dysfunction and ventricular arrhythmias. The combination of these poor prognostic signs was particularly ominous; this subset of post-MI patients (which represented only about 5% of the total population studied) had a >10-fold increased risk of dying.[22]

The relationship among noninvasive variables including the SAECG as prognostic tests after MI was explored in a study by Kuchar et al.[23] The study was formulated on the premise that the low specificity of the SAECG could be overcome by combining it with other test results. Of the 210 patients examined in this study, 15 patients experienced either sudden cardiac death or sustained VT. Three noninvasive tests provided results that were predictive of these arrhythmic events: an abnormal SAECG (odds ratio = 24), a low LVEF < 40% (odds ratio = 18), and complex ventricular ectopy on Holter (odds ratio = 8). All three were independently predictive by multivariate analysis. The probabilities of an arrhythmic event were amplified when the tests were used in combination, a legitimate endeavor given their independent predictive value. The likelihood of an arrhythmic event was quite low in the 14-month follow-up of the study cohort when either the Holter or the SAECG were normal, but markedly higher when both were positive. The event rate jumped from 0%–6% to >30% in the subset with both Holter and SAECG abnormal as shown in Figure 6.2. Similarly, the SAECG was analyzed in conjunction with the LVEF. The risk of an arrhythmic event increased from 0%–4% to 34% in patients with an LVEF < 40% who had an abnormal SAECG (Figure 6.3). The specificity was indeed

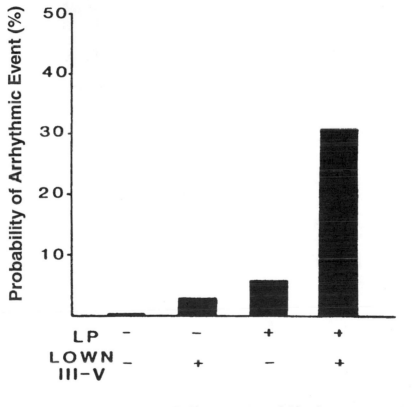

Figure 6.2. The predictive value, individually and in combination, of the results of SAECG-detected late potentials (LP) or prolonged filtered QRS duration, and Lown grade ventricular arrhythmia on Holter recording. (Reprinted with permission from JACC; Kuchar et al.[23])

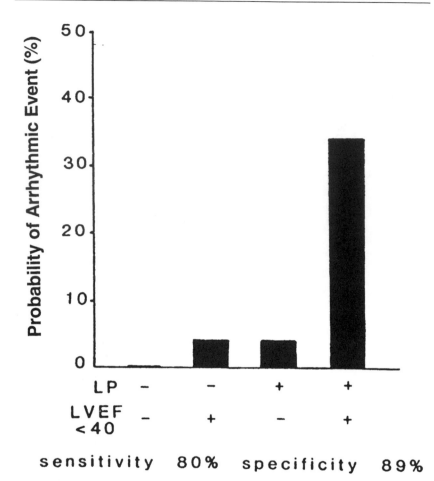

Figure 6.3. The predictive value, individually and in combination, of the results of SAECG-detected late potentials (LP) or prolonged filtered QRS duration, and reduced LVEF <40%. (Reprinted with permission from JACC; Kuchar et al.[23])

improved when using the SAECG in combination with these other tests, to a level approaching 90%, without a major loss of sensitivity.

These observations suggest that the SAECG can help identify which patients with severe left ventricular dysfunction or ventricular arrhythmia have the conduction characteristics required to sustain fatal arrhythmic events. Conversely, extensive ventricular damage or the presence of arrhythmic triggers are generally needed to initiate and perpetuate these dangerous arrhythmias.

Replacement with scar tissue of formerly healthy and functioning myocardial tissue is the hallmark of healed MI. The presence and extent of scar tissue is reflected noninvasively in the LVEF. However, specific electrical and pathological characteristics of the scar are closely tied to the expression of VT due to reentry and may explain the ability to use clinical tools with ejection fraction to predict arrhythmia. The interruption of normal cell-to-cell coupling of the ventricular myocardium creates the possibility of slowed ventricular conduction directly and by mechanisms such as anisotropy. Necrosis of myocardial cells and the subsequent scarring with fibrotic tissue provide the anatomic basis for these electrical sequelae. Specifically, the type of infarct border tissue is a critical determinant of conduction delay in sinus rhythm[24]; greater irregularity due to patchiness (scar tissue interposed between viable tissue) of healing is associated with greater conduction delay.

Similar clinical observations to those of Kuchar et al.[23] were made by Gomes and colleagues in 1987.[25] Using data derived from a prospective study of 102 patients, malignant ventricular arrhythmias (sustained VT, cardiac arrest, or sudden death) were predicted by the SAECG, Holter ECG, and LVEF. Quantitative SAECG values were strikingly different between patients who experienced an arrhythmia event (n=15) and those who did not (n=81); these patients had a longer filtered QRSd and low-amplitude signal, as well as a lower RMS voltage in the terminal 40 msec of the QRS. The SAECG provided the most sensitive and specific results among the three noninvasive tests examined. Utilizing combinations of two and three tests allowed more precise and powerful stratification, but these analyses were hampered by inadequate sample sizes. The Cox survivorship model identified the SAECG, LVEF, and nonsustained VT on Holter as predictors of ventricular arrhythmic events.

Another study[26] utilized early SAECG (on day 3 post-MI) in 159 patients and related arrhythmic events to SAECG results alone, and in combination with Holter obtained > 6 days post-MI. A late potential was present in 24% of patients, and 26% of these patients experienced an arrhythmic event in follow-up. Thus, the SAECG recorded early in the hospital phase after MI predicted life-threatening arrhythmic events in the months after MI. The successful use of early SAECG is of particular importance because hospital stays have progressively shortened due to improved patient prognosis and greater economic pressures. Thus, early risk stratification with the SAECG may be feasible and may even be helpful for decision-making regarding early hospital discharge. The combination of frequent ventricular ectopy on the Holter tape with an abnormal SAECG substantially augmented the positive predictive accuracy (to 62%) yet maintained sensitivity at a respectable level (73%).

A detailed analysis of the interaction among left ventricular function, spontaneous ventricular arrhythmia on Holter ECG, and the SAECG was performed by Steinberg et al.[4] This prospective study enrolled 182 patients in the convalescent period after acute MI. The presence of an abnormal SAECG result was not strongly related to the presence of left ventricular dysfunction. The LVEF was depressed (<0.40) in 45% of patients with an abnormal SAECG compared to 38% in patients with well preserved LVEF. The likelihood of an SAECG recording yielding a positive finding was a nonsignificant 1.33 times higher in patients with LVEF <0.40. The presence of ventricular arrhythmia on Holter was found in 35% of patients with an abnormal SAECG result and in 25% of patients with a normal SAECG. The likelihood of the SAECG recording showing an abnormality was a nonsignficant 1.57 times higher in patients with ventricular arrhythmia on Holter. Thus, the SAECG had a weak association with either low LVEF or Holter findings of ventricular arrhythmia.

Similar to findings of other contemporary studies, this investigation found that left ventricular function, Holter ECG detection of frequent or complex ventricular arrhythmia, and the SAECG findings were all significant predictors of arrhythmic events during follow-up. Multivariate analysis identified only the SAECG as an independent variable for predicting the development of a fatal or potentially fatal ventricular arrhythmia.

Various combinations of variables were explored to maximize the clinical value and utility of noninvasive screening (Table 6.1). Screening tests in general have two goals: identify or exclude high risk. In this study, individual tests performed suboptimally regardless of desired screening goal; the SAECG, however, had the best sensitivity. Tests used in combination performed much better and at levels where meaningful clinical decision making would result. For example, the absence of left ventricular dysfunction, Holter arrhythmia, and abnormal SAECG virtually excluded the development of dangerous ventricular arrhythmias after MI (negative predictive accuracy of 98%). The presence of both Holter arrhythmia and positive SAECG findings pinpointed a subgroup of post-MI patients (about 13% of total group) at extremely high risk. This subgroup had an event rate of 25% at 1 year and 60% at 2 years of follow-up, far greater than the remainder of the post-MI population. Figure

Table 6.1
Clinical Value of Noninvasive Testing of
Post-Myocardial Infarction Patients

Test	Sensitivity (%)	Specificity (%)	+ Predictive Accuracy (%)	− Predictive Accuracy (%)
LVEF < 0.40	57	61	12	94
+ Holter	44	73	13	93
+ SAECG	69	62	15	95
LVEF < 0.40 or + SAECG	86	39	12	97
+ Holter or + SAECG	75	47	13	95
LVEF < 0.40 or + Holter or + SAECG	93	31	11	98
LVEF < 0.40 and + Holter	21	85	12	92
LVEF < 0.40 and + SAECG	36	83	17	93
+ Holter and + SAECG	38	89	25	93
LVEF < 0.40 and + Holter and + SAECG	21	94	25	93

LVEF = left ventricular ejection fraction; SAECG = signal-averaged electrocardiogram.

6.4 demonstrates these observations in Kaplan-Meier survival plots. This level of risk warrants grave concern and intervention to the extent that medical knowledge permits. One might conclude that the SAECG detects conduction delay but the occurrence of sustained arrhythmia requires the presence of triggering ventricular complexes in many patients. Importantly, this analysis also highlights the clinical use of combination screening derived from the independence of test results and underlying pathophysiology.

The independent prognostic value of the SAECG has been hampered by drawing conclusions from the relatively small studies (and thus endpoints) performed at single institutions. Why is this important? If the SAECG is to be used as a screening test in clinical trials, as a surrogate endpoint in clinical investigation, and as a test guiding clinical practice, it must be shown with a high degree of confidence that the SAECG is providing unique clinical data in terms of risk stratification. Despite the logic and uniqueness of measuring ventricular conduction, it is not inconceivable that the data provided by the SAECG overlaps with that provided by other readily available and well-established tests, i.e., LVEF and the Holter ECG. A review

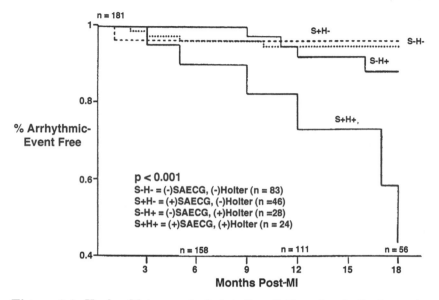

Figure 6.4. Kaplan-Meier survival plot of prediction of arrhythmic events after myocardial infarction (post-MI) by results of SAECG and Holter recording. (Reprinted with permission from American Journal of Cardiology; Steinberg et al.[4])

of several studies[27] showed that the SAECG results often did not provide risk data independent of these clinical tests if interpretations were restricted to the individual trials in the published literature (Figure 6.5). In meta-analyses of these published trials,[23,25-27] which used these noninvasive screening tests to predict risk after MI, it was clearly established from the pooled analyses that the SAECG provided independent risk information. From three studies[23,25,27] that followed almost 500 patients, the SAECG predicted a sixfold increase in risk independent of LVEF. From four studies[23,25-27] that followed more than 650 patients, the SAECG predicted an eightfold increase in risk of arrhythmic events independent of ventricular arrhythmia on Holter ECG. A recent Cardiac Arrhythmia Suppression Trial (CAST) of over 1000 patients largely confirmed these relationships[28] although the results may have been tainted by use of CAST antiarrhythmic drugs in some patients, selection of a low risk population, and inconsistent performance of noninvasive screening tests at participating centers.

The ultimate development of sudden cardiac death is the result of a complex interplay of several factors pivotal to the pathophysiology of sustained ventricular tachyarrhythmias in the setting of coro-

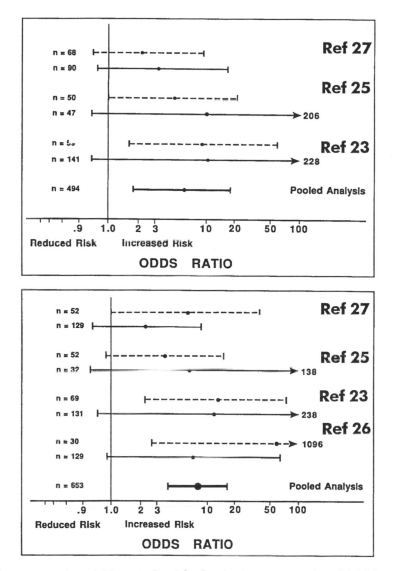

Figure 6.5. Top. Odds ratio for risk of arrhythmic event when SAECG was abnormal in three prospective studies with left ventricular ejection fraction (LVEF) stratified at 0.40. Dashed lines represent LVEF <0.40 and solid lines LVEF ≥0.40. Bold line is pooled results. **Bottom**. Odds ratio for risk of arrhythmic event when SAECG was abnormal in four prospective studies with Holter results to presence or absence of frequent or repetitive ventricular arrhythmia. Dashed lines represent presence and solid lines absence of ventricular arrhythmia on Holter. Bold line is pooled results. (Reprinted with permission from American Journal of Cardiology; Steinberg et al.[4])

nary heart disease. Clues to the complexity of the pathogenesis of sudden cardiac death come from several different experimental models and also from observations in clinical trials and investigations. It is apparent that alterations in autonomic tone that follow the aftermath of MI can affect arrhythmogenesis; heightened cardiac sympathetic tone is proarrhythmic while parasympathetic tone is antiarrhythmic. The degree of regularity of the cardiac impulse originating in the sinus node is highly sensitive to autonomic input and provides a handy and accurate measure of resting and dynamic autonomic tone. This analysis, known as heart rate variability, can be done in the time or frequency domains, and has been shown to predict both cardiac and arrhythmic death after MI.

A recent prospective study[29] of 416 patients integrated this new noninvasive measure with previous tests known to be predictive of postinfarction arrhythmic events. In contrast to the SAECG, heart rate variability was significantly (but weakly) related to the LVEF and frequency of ventricular arrhythmia on Holter. Patients with reduced heart rate variability were more than twice as likely to have an abnormal SAECG: 37% versus 16%. In a mean follow-up approaching 2 years, there were 24 arrhythmic events.

The heart rate variability was markedly reduced and the presence of late potentials much higher in the patients who experienced an arrhythmic event. Limited by the sample size, it was apparent that patients were far more likely to develop postinfarction arrhythmic events if any one of several noninvasive tests were abnormal but in particular the heart rate variability analysis and the SAECG (Table 6.2). Interestingly, these patient characteristics also predicted cardiac death. All tests were associated with low positive predictive accuracy (<20%) and were evaluated in various combinations to improve risk stratification. The combination of low heart rate variability and late potentials was a particularly ominous finding; the risk of an arrhythmic event increased 18-fold. Of all tested combinations, the presence of low heart rate variability and late potentials maintained a sensitivity >50%.

The presence of abnormal autonomic tone may facilitate the development of ventricular arrhythmia in patients susceptible as indicated by the SAECG. Evolving technology will soon permit the simultaneous recording of all ECG-derived indices: ventricular arrhythmia, heart rate variability, and SAECG as well as even newer markers of risk such as QT dispersion. In the near future, a single recording will be highly informative, efficient, and cost-effective.

Table 6.2
Ranked Univariate Relation of Variables to
Arrhythmic Events in 416 Patients

	Log-Rank Analysis	Cox Proportional Hazards Regression Coefficient	Proportional Hazards Chi-Square	Relative Risk (95% CI)
Heart rate variability <20 msec	0.0000	3.48	55.7	32.4 (7.6–138)
Ventricular ectopic beats >10/hour	0.0000	1.61	15.37	4.98 (2.2–11.1)
Repetitive ventricular forms	0.0000	1.58	15.01	4.89 (2.2–10.0)
Mean RR interval <750 msec	0.0000	1.59	13.57	4.93 (2.1–11.5)
Late positive potentials	0.0000	1.88	19.8	6.53 (2.9–14.9)
Killip class ≥2	0.0181	0.96	5.18	2.61 (1.1–5.6)
Left ventricular ejection fraction <40%	0.0191	0.93	5.12	2.53 (1.1–5.6)

Exercise testing, age >65 years, site of infarction, or Q wave infarction had no univariate relation to arrhythmic events. The initial relation between variables and arrhythmic events is expressed as the Kaplan-Meier product estimate of the survival function (log-rank) multivariate analysis; the relative risk is calculated from the Cox analysis. CI = confidence interval. (Reprinted with permission from JACC; Farrell TG, et al.[29])

Signal-Averaged Electrocardiogram Variables or Components as Risk Predictors

The interrelationships among noninvasive variables and among SAECG variables have important implications for their clinical use, either singly or in combination. For example, Gomes et al.[3] examined the presence of late potentials based on the high-pass filter frequency used in SAECG analysis. Two commonly used filter cutoffs were 25 Hz and 40 Hz. Overall, the proportion of abnormal SAECG results was nearly identical regardless of high-pass filtering. About 10% of the sample analyzed had discordant results between the two analyses. Thus, in general, results are similar regardless of filter frequency used; when results are discrepant it usually is based on minor changes in the terminal portion of the QRS.

In the study by Steinberg et al.,[4] both V40 and low-amplitude signal were not predictive of arrhythmic events as univariate variables and were not independent of total filtered (at 40 Hz) QRS duration (fQRS). The fQRS was highly predictive on its own; there was a threefold increased risk of an arrhythmic event when the fQRS was prolonged. The fQRS as a risk variable is probably best viewed as a continuous variable since any effort to dichotomize the data is always arbitrary. The fQRS is a strongly related risk of arrhythmic events as a continuous variable and is plotted in Figure 6.6. When the fQRS was <100 msec, the risk was negligible. The risk increased to about 9% when the fQRS was at the upper limit of most normal ranges. When the fQRS exceeded 120 msec, the risk was >10%, and jumped to 31% in the small group of patients whose fQRS was >130 msec. The curvilinear relationship between fQRS and arrhythmic risk as shown in Figure 6.6 is important to keep in mind when interpreting SAECG results. Clearly, the longer the fQRS, the

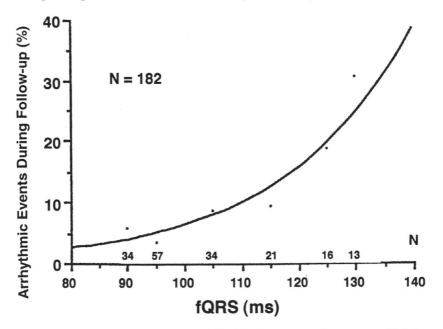

Figure 6.6. Relation of risk of arrhythmic events after myocardial infarction and the value of the filtered QRS duration (fQRS). (Reprinted with permission from American Journal of Cardiology; Steinberg et al.[4])

greater the risk, and the risk becomes remarkably high when the fQRS is uncommonly prolonged. In a multivariate analysis of clinical and SAECG variables, it was discovered that the total QRSd when filtered at 40 Hz had the strongest relation to outcome,[3] corroborating the above described findings.

Technical and Clinical Limitations to the Use of the Signal-Averaged Electrocardiogram after Myocardial Infarction

Technical factors are at issue in risk prediction as well, and have been reviewed in previous chapters. Foremost among them are the recording sensitivity for all of ventricular activation, timing of abnormal segments relative to the predominant deflection of the QRS, inability to differentiate conduction delay due to BBB from myocardial delay, and inability to record transient or changing myocardial signals.

It has been a common observation for the subset of post-MI patients with inferior MI to have a higher prevalence of SAECG abnormalities than patients with anterior MI. Because patients with anterior MI are more likely to have ventricular tachyarrhythmias than patients with inferior MI, we now see one of the problems inherent in time domain SAECG analysis. The posterior septum (part of the inferior distribution) is activated last in the normal sequence of ventricular activation, while the anterior septum and anterior wall are activated early. Thus delays in conduction arising from the inferior and posterior walls are more likely to extend (in time) beyond the depolarization of the remainder of the LV and thus produce a late potential, whereas the delays present in the anterior wall are more likely to get "buried" within the QRS and not outlast the bulk of LV activation and not create a late potential. Therefore, we would predict that sensitivity for VT/VF is lower in anterior MI and specificity for VT/VF is lower in inferior MI. Despite these handicaps, there is a great deal of overlap and the SAECG is still capable of predicting arrhythmic events in patients with MI. This problem cannot be overcome with standard SAECG analysis.

Based on this physiological disadvantage, one would predict high sensitivity and low specificity for arrhythmic events in patients with inferior MI. In contrast, patients with anterior MI would be expected to have lower sensitivity and greater specificity for arrhythmic events. In one analysis,[3] in patients with inferior MI, the sensitivity was 100% and specificity only 50% whereas better predictions were made in patients with anterior MI in whom the sensitivity was 75% and specificity was 80%. Readers should exercise caution in the interpretation of these subgroup analyses because groups were small and thus subject to very wide confidence intervals. Large trials or meta-analyses would clarify this problematic issue.

All of the aforementioned prospective studies grouped together all presumed "arrhythmic events," including patients who had sustained VT with those who had documented cardiac arrest due to VF and those who had sudden, often unwitnessed, death. Because the electrophysiological substrate may differ between stable VT and unstable VT,[24] it may be more appropriate to examine SAECG variables based on more specific arrhythmic outcomes in prospective studies. Unfortunately, the small number of arrhythmia-specific events in all published trials makes this analysis problematic. One group[30] has raised the possibility that important differences in SAECG variables may exist for the prediction of sustained VT relative to sudden death. This is in agreement with simultaneous endocardial mapping and SAECG studies that contrasted cardiac arrest (VT) patients. The patients with VT had more extensive late conduction abnormalities on direct and SAECG recordings, indicating more extensive arrhythmogenic substrate.[31] Further work will be needed to fully address this concern.

The discussion in the preceding sections makes it abundantly clear that the SAECG has predictive power for arrhythmic events in the recovery period after MI. It should be recognized that like all prognostic tests, the ability to predict VTs and sudden cardiac death is inherently limited by a fundamental lack of a comprehensive understanding regarding the initial development of the clinical event. In addition one must accept that our ability to define the clinical event as arrhythmic in origin is also greatly hampered both by a lack of electrocardiographic documentation in many instances and by the fact that VT or VF may simply be the final common pathway of demise in some patients resulting from another primary process. The cause of death in the patient after MI may result from recurrent ischemia/infarction, congestive heart failure, cardiac rupture, electromechanical dissociation, bradyarrhythmias and asystole, and related noncardiac conditions such as pulmonary embolus and cerebrovascular accident. Assignment of the cause of death in the individual patient is a difficult, if not artificial, process because of the complexity and overlap of mechanisms involved.

Interaction of Invasive Risk Stratification with Programmed Ventricular Stimulation and the Signal-Averaged Electrocardiogram

Arising from the limitations of risk stratification using noninvasive methods, attempts were made to use programmed ventricular stimulation to predict morbid or fatal arrhythmic events after MI. Like the SAECG, the induction of sustained monomorphic VT was thought to represent a specific indication of the presence of arrhythmic substrate for VT. However, the actual completion and perpetuation of the reentrant circuit was construed as a logical marker for the later clinical development of VT. This section will not attempt to fully discuss the merits and problems with EPS used for these purposes, but will instead concentrate on the interrelationships between EPS and the SAECG. In concept, this interaction can take two forms: the SAECG can be used to predict which patients will have electrically inducible VT (as distinct from clinical or spontaneous VT) and thus screen for the EPS, or the SAECG can be used in conjunction with EPS if these results provide independent information.

The first group to explore these possibilities was Breithardt et al.[32] This was the first of a series of publications by this group examining the correlation between late potentials, inducible VT, and arrhythmic events. The patients studied were those referred for coronary angiography after MI who were then also tested with the SAECG and EPS. Thus the samples included in this prospective analysis were not necessarily representative of unselected individuals in the convalescent phase of MI. The technique of SAECG used by Breithardt's group was described in the previous section and has distinct limitations but nonetheless can provide visual evidence of late potential activity.

Late potentials were identified in 45% of the 132 patients studied in this investigation, with late potentials of the longest duration present in 16%. As reported in several other studies, patients with inferior MI were more likely to have late potentials on SAECG. Programmed ventricular stimulation produced repetitive ventricular responses in a large segment of the total group (46%), but only 21% had a sustained arrhythmia (VT or VF) induced. There was no difference in the induction of arrhythmia relative to site of MI.

The nature of the endpoint of EPS at that time has evolved so that induction of arrhythmia that is not sustained is now often considered nonspecific (in part, on the basis of studies like this one); thus the interpretation of this study is hampered. It is evident that patients were more likely to have sustained VT at rates <270 bpm if a late potential was present (36%), than if a late potential was absent (21%). This VT EPS endpoint was critical because one/four of these patients went on to present with spontaneous VT whereas none of the patients with other EPS endpoints or no inducible arrhythmia had spontaneous VT. While the EPS had predicted all spontaneous VT events (sensitivity 100%), SAECG fared slightly less well (sensitivity 78%). The risk of spontaneous VT was also related to the duration of the late potential. Neither test predicted sudden cardiac death, but there were very few endpoints.

Using the data in this study, the authors suggested a stepwise approach to risk stratification. The first step was the SAECG, which identified most, but not all, who would develop spontaneous VT. However, the low predictive accuracy of a positive test could be doubled (from 11% to 20%) with the second step in this approach, namely the EPS. Importantly, this step did not miss any patients who later had sustained VT because of its higher sensitivity as well as specificity.

In one of the most comprehensive studies of risk prediction after MI, Richards[33] exposed 361 patients to a battery of tests, both invasive and noninvasive. Not all patients underwent all tests, but most patients underwent EPS, SAECG, nuclear radionuclide angiogram, 24-hour ambulatory ECG, and exercise testing. The SAECG was analyzed as an unfiltered three-lead recording, and the duration of ventricular activation (earliest on any lead to latest on any lead) was prolonged if >120 msec. Terminal QRS measurements were not utilized. Patients were followed for more than 2 years and did not receive routine beta-blocker therapy.

There were 34 deaths during follow-up, of which eight were sudden, and there were nine patients who survived episodes of sustained VT or VF. The risk of either sudden cardiac death or VT/VF was increased when patients had inducible VT at EPS (relative risk = 15), reduced LVEF (relative risk = 4.8), or abnormal SAECG (relative risk = 4.4). Other noninvasive tests did not contribute to risk prediction. With multivariate analysis, only inducible VT and LVEF made significant contributions and the EPS was clearly the critical variable for any possible model. For cardiac death (including death due to arrhythmia, ischemia, and heart failure), the SAECG was the most powerful predictor (relative risk = 7), followed by EPS (relative risk = 5.6) and LVEF (relative risk = 5.2); all three were independent predictors with multivariate analysis.

In an earlier study, these same investigators examined the overlap of results between SAECG and EPS.[21] Interestingly, in this cohort, these tests had similar predictive values, but the correspondence between tests was imperfect. Of the 80 patients with delayed potentials, nine patients (11%) had inducible VT. Although VT inducibility was uncommon even in this group, it was still far more frequent than in the much larger group without delayed potentials in whom VT was induced in only 4 of 226 patients (2%). However, using the SAECG to screen for EPS would have missed 4 of the 13 patients with VT (30%), a substantial false negative finding. Because of this incomplete overlap between SAECG and EPS, more data will be needed to demonstrate that the noninvasive SAECG can predict with accuracy the invasive EPS results in this particular setting.

These data indicate that EPS provides the most important information regarding risk stratification. However, EPS is not universally available, is expensive, and has a small risk. It clearly cannot be the procedure of choice unless and until the results of EPS are specifically needed for risk modification because of the need to focus on those at greatest risk or to learn the characteristics of the potential VT circuit. There is currently no therapeutic intervention that mandates routine EPS. The SAECG, along with LVEF, emerged as the most important markers of risk in the study by Richards et al.[33] Interestingly, this study found that the SAECG had a high specificity and intermediate sensitivity. It is likely that the technique of SAECG recording and analysis accounts for this observation and underlines the fact that a simple SAECG measurement is potent and does not necessitate other quantitative maneuvers.

A recent comprehensive prospective investigation[34] further examined the role of both noninvasive and invasive risk stratification. This study provided additional and confirmatory data to those described above. It was a large program, enrolling over 300 patients at a cardiac rehabilitation center approximately 3 weeks after MI; bear in mind that this method of patient recruitment may introduce selection bias. A major strength of this study was the use of a full battery of noninvasive tests with very few patients who did not undergo the complete testing process. The authors then selected patients to undergo programmed ventricular stimulation based on the presence of at least two abnormal noninvasive test results. One drawback of the study was the nonuse of beta-blockers during the testing process and the sparing use of beta-blockers during follow-up despite the proven benefit of beta-blockers on arrhythmic mortality in patients after MI.

As in several previous studies, the results of SAECG (especially the filtered QRS duration) were predictive of the 19 arrhythmic events in the cohort, independent of the other noninvasive variables that were also predictive (LVEF, nonsustained VT on Holter, and heart rate variability index). About one quarter of the total patient group was preselected to have EPS, but one third of this subgroup declined participation. Unfortunately, this large group excluded from EPS may further bias the study results. With these limitations in mind, EPS was far superior to any noninvasive test at identifying the patients who subsequently experienced serious arrhythmic events. Of the 20 patients with inducible VT <270 bpm, 13 went on to experience an arrhythmic event compared to only 1 of 27 without inducible VT <270 bpm (relative risk = 17). The positive predictive value for arrhythmic events of 65% is much higher than one sees even when multiple noninvasive tests are used in combination. These authors also recommended a two-staged screening process. The first step was noninvasive assessment to be followed by EPS when at least two noninvasive variables were abnormal. This approach was associated with very few false negative results yet provided accurate identification of high-risk patients.

The relevance of using this strategy, or for that matter any noninvasive strategy, to guide the initiation of antiarrhythmic medical therapy is unproven at best and hazardous in many instances. Future studies must clarify the complementary role of noninvasive and invasive screening strategies as they specifically relate to treatment, not simply risk, before any recommendations can be made regarding risk modification. In the next few years, we are likely to learn about the role of amiodarone and other class III antiarrhythmic drugs, as well as the implantable cardioverter-defibrillator (ICD), as secondary preventive measures. Integration of optimal risk assessment schemas with treatment strategies will be a major challenge for electrophysiologists and clinical cardiologists. Many issues will come to bear on this process, such as intrinsic test value, cost considerations, and test and manpower availability.

Although the EPS is the single best predictor of spontaneous VT and sudden cardiac death, noninvasive risk prediction with SAECG, Holter, LVEF, and perhaps newer modalities such as heart rate variability and T-wave alternans, has clear-cut and important clinical relevance.

The Clinical Utility of the Signal-Averaged Electrocardiogram in the Thrombolytic Era

Attempts at reperfusion of occluded coronary arteries, most commonly with thrombolytic therapy, have evolved to standard treatment for acute MI. This approach, with a variety of regimens, has reduced cardiac mortality. Because most of the studies that addressed the value of the SAECG for stratifying post-MI risk were performed before thrombolytic therapy became the norm, one may legitimately raise several questions. Does thrombolytic therapy, or its intended result (patency of the infarct artery), alter the likelihood of developing an abnormal SAECG? Is the SAECG still of value in predicting arrhythmic risk when patients are routinely treated with thrombolytic therapy? Several recent efforts provide solid data relevant to these issues.

There have been several uncontrolled studies that observed a significant decrease in the frequency and severity of SAECG abnormality in patients after thrombolysis[35-38] and even greater improvement (sometimes striking) in patients in whom the infarct artery was shown to be patent at subsequent angiography.[35-41] Observation of the SAECG during administration of thrombolytic therapy has revealed substantial reduction in the frequency of abnormal recording after successful reperfusion but no reduction with persistent occlusion.[42] However, despite the concordance of findings, these trials were regarded with caution because of the absence of prospective, randomized, or placebo-controlled series.

More recently, we published the only prospective, randomized, and placebo-controlled study of the effect of thrombolysis on the SAECG.[43] As part of a multicenter investigation of the benefit of late administration of thrombolytic therapy, it was unequivocally demonstrated that the SAECG is improved when reperfusion therapy was administered between 6 and 24 hours after onset of symptoms. The fQRS was shortened and the proportion of patients with a prolonged fQRS was reduced in the treated group of 150 patients compared to the placebo group of 160 patients. It is noteworthy that the improvement in SAECG was limited to patients who presented with ST elevation on their ECG. In this group of 185 patients, the frequency of SAECG abnormality was halved, a striking reduction as shown in Figure 6.7. In those without ST elevation, no improvement was seen. Moreover, there was a consistent leftward shift of the plot of fQRS duration to less pronounced prolongation throughout the range of measured values (Figure 6.8). These observations sug-

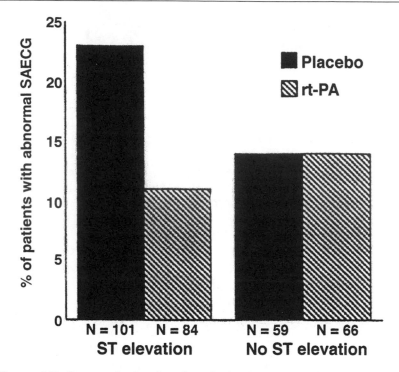

Figure 6.7. Bar graph showing the relation between qualifying ECG and the effect of recombinant tissue-type plasminogen activator (rt-PA) on frequency of abnormal SAECG. Administration of rt-PA reduced the incidence of abnormal SAECG in patients with ST elevation (p=0.011) but not in patients whose ECG did not have ST elevation. (Reprinted with permission from Circulation; Steinberg et al.[43])

gested that reperfusion of a totally occluded infarct artery, even relatively late after onset of symptoms of MI, leads to a more stable electrical substrate, which likely reflects a meaningful, if not substantial, mechanism of mortality benefit.

Although the benefit of medical reperfusion on the SAECG is clear, the possible advantage of more delayed mechanical reperfusion is less settled. One small study[44] suggested that angioplasty of a previously occluded infarct artery can cause resolution of late potentials during short-term follow-up. A larger study[45] found no such benefit although another intriguing observation was made. When the occluded infarct artery was successfully opened, the absence of SAECG abnormality predicted improvement in wall motion in the infarct zone. The SAECG may thus be used to indicate viability of infarct zone myocardium but only if these initial observations are confirmed.

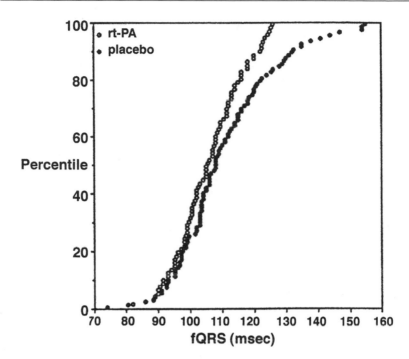

Figure 6.8. The proportional distribution of patients, according to treatment assignment, relative to total filtered QRS duration (fQRS) in patients with ST elevation prior to qualification for treatment. There is a consistent leftward shift in the recombinant tissue-type plasminogen activator (rt-PA) patients that becomes attenuated at long fQRS values. More patients had less prolonged fQRS throughout the fQRS range if treated with rt-PA. (Reprinted with permission from Circulation; Steinberg et al.[43])

The ultimate expression of VTs after MI is a complex and dynamic process. Although conduction delay as measured by the SAECG is a determinant of arrhythmia formation, an appropriate balance between conduction and recovery of excitability must exist for reentry to occur. These electrical properties may in turn be modulated by infarct pathology, ischemia, left ventricular volume, and nervous system innervation. These processes are all potentially related to the presence, timing, and degree of reperfusion. One such interrelationship—that between late potential formation and ventricular dilation—was carefully examined by Zaman et al.[46] In this study, early phase late potentials (first week post-MI) predicted the development of ventricular enlargement several weeks later. The authors hypothesized that early myocardial cell slippage is responsible for both early conduction delay and later ventricular dilation.

Table 6.3 summarizes the published experience with use of the SAECG for risk prediction after MI when substantial segments of the clinical population have received thrombolytic therapy. The study populations have not uniformly received thrombolytic therapy but instead were treated on clinical grounds or part of nonrandomized clinical trials. Although many patients remain ineligible or untreated with thrombolytic therapy in contemporary practice, these studies may still reasonably reflect current post-MI patients.

Several general observations are worthy of emphasis. Mortality post-infarction continues to fall due to many factors including thrombolytic therapy. Arrhythmic events parallel this trend as exemplified in these studies; arrhythmic event rates are substantially less than those reported in the earlier studies of SAECG. Studies of other arrhythmic endpoints, such as inducible VT at EPS, also show similar findings.[47] Because of a low event rate, risk stratification tests face a more difficult burden (based on Bayes' theorem) and prospective studies become more difficult to interpret due to the broader confidence intervals that are inevitably present.

The overall incidence of positive SAECG results is lower than previously described, presumably reduced by the component of the study population that received thrombolytic therapy. It can be seen that all studies showed an increased risk of arrhythmic events when the SAECG was abnormal, even in populations where as many as

Table 6.3
Prognostic Value of the Post-MI SAECG in the Thrombolytic Era

Ref. No.	Total #/ #Thrombo-lytic Rx	SAECG Day No.	No. of (+) SAECG	Duration of F/U (mos)	Arrhythmic Events (total group)		Prognostic Value of (+) SAECG				
					SCD	VT-S	Sens	Spec	(+)PV	(−)PV	RR*
38	174/106	26±10	41 (24%)	14±8	4	4	75	82	18	98	13.0
48	331/130	5-11	48 (15%)	20	12	13	48	88	25	95	6.9
49	301/205	14	61 (20%)	13	11	2	64	81	11	98	7.5
51	173/88	10-20	41 (24%)	12±5	7	2	56	78	12	97	4.4
50	787/363**	5-30	97 (12%)	10±3	31	2	90	61	21	98	13.0

* Uncorrected
** Includes angioplasty in same patients
F/U = follow-up; MI = myocardial infarction; PV = predictive value; RR = relative risk; Rx = therapy; SAECG = signal-averaged ECG; SCD = sudden cardiac death; Sens = sensitivity; Spec = specificity; VT-S = sustained VT; Ref = reference.

two thirds received thrombolytic therapy. One study[38] examined the subgroup that was treated with thrombolytic therapy, and within this subgroup the SAECG predicted arrhythmic events. However, Malik and colleagues[48] found that the SAECG had greater predictive accuracy in the group that did not receive streptokinase; these conclusions should be cautiously interpreted because patients in this subgroup were at higher risk.

The issue of timing of SAECG and its relation to prediction of arrhythmic events was examined by McClements et al.[49] Serial SAECGs were recorded at 48 hours, at day 6, and at hospital discharge. Only the final recording proved to be statistically significant. With shorter hospital stays becoming increasingly prevalent and with thrombolytic therapy routine, the issue of appropriate timing of SAECG for risk stratification will need to be revisited in larger contemporary studies that have the power to discriminate between several SAECG recordings per patient.

Multivariate analysis in the study with the largest number of patients treated with thrombolysis[50] revealed a potent independent association between SAECG findings and arrhythmic events. This study did not include coronary angiographic data. When Hohnloser et al.[51] also evaluated the independence of SAECG risk prediction, it was discovered that although the SAECG was a univariate predictor, it was not independent of the patency of infarct artery on the coronary angiogram.

Sustained coronary perfusion appears to be a critical factor in the development of late serious arrhythmias after MI. Specific electrical properties of the ventricular myocardium may be modulated by a number of processes that are directly or indirectly affected by timely reperfusion during acute MI and also by sustained perfusion in the chronic phase of MI healing. These interdependent myocardial factors include infarct pathology, integrity of the infarct border zone, left ventricular remodeling and volume, and sympathetic innervation. Ventricular conduction, assessed by the SAECG, has a strong relation to the patency of the infarct artery; in patients exposed to pharmacological thrombolytic therapy, the incidence of late potentials has been low in patients with patent infarct artery, and is several times more common when the infarct artery was occluded.[35,36,39,40,49] Early timing of thrombolytic therapy may not be as critical as the ultimate development of patency and sustained and complete perfusion of the culprit coronary artery.[52] The ability of thrombolytic therapy to accelerate the rate of and increase the proportion of patients with infarct artery patency explains the lower incidence of SAECG abnormalities as well as a lower risk of mortality; these two outcomes are likely interrelated. Large-scale clinical trials will be needed to definitively explore this issue.

There is clearly an interaction among successful reperfusion, patency of the infarct artery, and the development of arrhythmic substrate exemplified by the SAECG. Among noninvasive tests, the SAECG retains its predictive power for arrhythmic events. The combined use of angiographic and noninvasive results will need additional study in much larger populations than have been published to date. However, cardiac catheterization is not yet routinely performed and unless there are accurate noninvasive predictors of infarct artery patency, physicians must still rely on data that are easily and regularly obtainable.

Evolution of the Signal-Averaged Electrocardiogram in the First Year after Myocardial Infarction

Whether hospital discharge is the optimal time for SAECG recording and whether there is a clinically meaningful evolution of the SAECG after hospital discharge were the subjects of several prospective investigations.

In one such study,[53] 192 patients were assessed serially, at five time points in the first year after MI. The most important finding was that SAECG parameters did not change throughout this time frame and that there was moderate to strong correlation between values at follow-up relative to the initial SAECG at hospital discharge (Figure 6.9). The number of patients with abnormal results remained relatively constant throughout follow-up. The vast majority of patients remained categorized in a similar way at each recording time; however, 10-20% of patients with early abnormal results "normalized" for at least one recording later in their course.

Other studies have suggested that the prevalence of late potentials may fall during follow-up, but these observations may be strongly influenced by technical issues. The SAECG is highly reproducible, but small changes in SAECG variables may occur and appear to change the overall results when the tracings were borderline to start with. For this reason, examining the SAECG variables as continuous data is much more meaningful than analysis with the SAECG as categorical. The Verzoni study[53] presents their results in this manner and thus has the most compelling contribution on this subject. Consistent with this assumption was the observation made by Kuchar et al.[54] that patients with greater degrees of SAECG

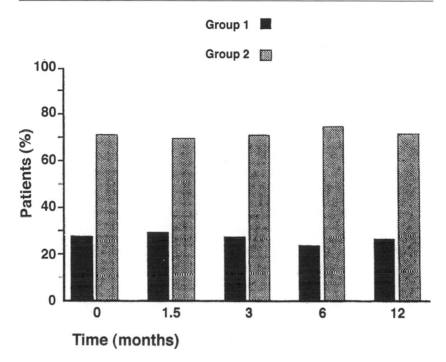

Figure 6.9. Serial results of SAECG after MI. Group I (n=62) represents patients with abnormal SAECG (two of three criteria) at hospital discharge and group 2 (n=158) represents patients with normal SAECG. (Reprinted with permission from PACE; Verzoni et al.[53])

abnormality were less likely to lose late potentials than patients with minimal abnormalities.

If in fact there is a tendency for the SAECG to change over time, especially toward a less prolonged and abnormal result[54-56] in some patients, despite the exaggeration of results by the technical issues raised in the preceding discussion, there is scientific rationale. Experimental support for a time dependence to conduction abnormality as measured with the SAECG exists and is consistent. We and others have shown that the prolongation of filtered QRSd is variable in the days following a canine model of MI, yet the risk of VT remains closely and temporally associated with SAECG results.[57,58] Pathologic changes as a result of healing, such as reestablishment of intercellular connections or resolution of ischemia, may play a role. On the other hand, when new bona fide abnormalities develop late after MI, an unusual occurrence in the absence of an intercurrent event, they may result from replacement of necrotic tissue with scar or an interaction with ischemia[41] and infarct artery patency. Similar temporal variability of results has been seen with VT inducibility in the days and weeks after MI.

When looked at prospectively, the timing of SAECG has influenced its capability as a prognostic test. Most[55,56,58] but not all[56] studies concluded that the best prediction was obtained from the predischarge SAECG compared to earlier or later recordings.

The bottom line on this subject is that there is compelling scientific and practical justification to perform the SAECG at the time of hospital discharge to optimally perform risk stratification.

Predicting Inducibility of Sustained Ventricular Tachycardia in Patients with Nonsustained Ventricular Tachycardia

The detection of nonsustained VT on ECG, telemetry recording, or Holter ECG is associated with adverse outcome. This association, limited to those with ventricular dysfunction, appears to be present whether the nonsustained VT is recorded in the convalescent phase of an acute event, e.g., MI, or during the chronic follow-up of patients with significant left ventricular dysfunction. Although nonsustained VT is viewed with grave concern, the management of these patients is as yet uncertain. Several multicenter trials are under way and their results should clarify the appropriate strategy to use in these patients. Most of these studies will use the EPS to refine risk prediction in the larger population of patients with nonsustained VT. This strategy is based on the premise that the results of EPS, chiefly the induction of sustained monomorphic VT, provide highly accurate risk stratification information that cannot be obtained by noninvasive means. In a study by Wilber et al.,[59] the patients with inducible VT that could not be suppressed by antiarrhythmic drugs had exceedingly high risk during follow-up; approximately 35% died suddenly during follow-up. This heightened event rate stood in contrast to either patients with suppressible VT or those with no inducible VT, both of whom had sudden death rates of approximately 5% during follow-up.

If EPS is the selected approach to management of the patient with nonsustained VT, it is unclear if all patients need be studied or if it is more efficient, clinically prudent, and cost-effective to perform EPS on prescreened subgroups. Several studies have examined the relationship of a variety of clinical and noninvasive variables to inducibility of VT and none, other than ejection fraction, has proven useful.

The SAECG has been studied for this purpose as well. In 1987, Buxton et al.[60] examined 43 patients referred over a 7-year period for EPS. Only 27 patients were asymptomatic; 13 patients had prior undiagnosed syncope. All participants exhibited ≥1 episode of non-sustained VT after acute MI, with an average longest duration of nonsustained VT of 15 complexes. In this study, comparisons were made among patients with nonsustained VT, patients with MI and infrequent ventricular arrhythmias and no nonsustained VT, and patients with documented sustained VT.

In the 43 patients with nonsustained VT, 22 had inducible sustained VT, a high rate undoubtedly influenced by the referred and symptomatic bias of the patient group. The analyses of this study focused on the differences of SAECG results in patients with inferior wall MI (n=29) compared to patients with anterior wall MI (n=14). Patients with inferior wall MI who had inducible sustained VT (n=16) had more fQRS prolongation and lower terminal voltages than their counterparts (n=13) without inducible sustained VT. In contrast, 14 patients with anterior wall MI demonstrated no differences in either SAECG measurement when the six patients with inducible VT were compared with the eight patients with a negative EPS. Nonetheless, both inferior wall MI and anterior wall MI patients exhibited a gradient of SAECG values from the least abnormal in patients without nonsustained VT to the greatest degree of abnormality in patients presenting with sustained VT. Patients with spontaneous nonsustained VT had intermediate SAECG results. These results are summarized in Figure 6.10.

Although the results of SAECG correlated with the EPS findings only in patients with inferior wall MI, it is likely that the small number of anterior wall MI patients with inducible sustained VT precluded a meaningful exploration of this issue. This study supported the hypothesis that, in at least some post-MI patients, SAECG may be useful as a predictor of inducible VT in high-risk patients identified by the presence of nonsustained VT. In fact, in patients with inferior wall MI, none of the seven patients without prolonged fQRS duration had inducible VT.

In a study of 105 heterogeneous patients, a similar analysis was performed.[61] However, the study population also included a large number of subjects with prolonged symptoms, such as syncope, which may have represented an episode of undiagnosed spontaneous sustained VT and thus overestimated the incidence of sustained VT

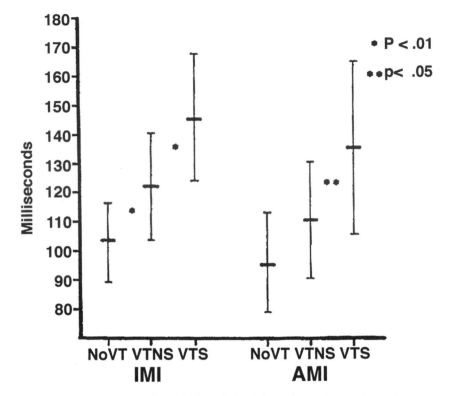

Figure 6.10. Relationship of filtered QRS duration to type of spontaneous ventricular arrhythmia and infarct location. VTNS = patients with nonsustained VT. (Reprinted with permission from American Journal of Cardiology; Buxton et al.[60])

in this population. The analysis revealed that those patients with inducible sustained monomorphic VT, 21% of the total group, were characterized by a history of syncope, a lower ejection fraction, and the presence of an abnormal SAECG. The differences in the SAECG results across patient groups were rather striking. For example, the fQRS duration was more than 20 msec longer in the sustained VT group, and late potentials were identified at least three times more commonly than in the groups with either sustained VF or no inducible arrhythmia. The sensitivity of the SAECG for inducible VT ranged between 64% and 73%, and the specificity ranged between 71% and 89%, depending on SAECG definition. Interestingly, the SAECG was as likely to be abnormal in the patients with coronary artery disease (25%) as those with idiopathic dilated cardiomyopathy (23%). Furthermore, the predictive accuracy was similar in these two groups. In a multivariate analysis, SAECG had the strongest association with inducible VT. However, the results of EPS and SAECG were not completely concordant; the SAECG misidentified 16% of the study patients based on EPS results.

In a smaller study[62] of 53 patients, about one quarter of whom had previous syncope, the SAECG was also found to predict inducible VT. In this study, only two extrastimuli were delivered during programmed ventricular stimulation, which likely altered the frequency of VT induction. In the 22 patients with abnormal SAECG recordings, 55% had inducible sustained or nonsustained monomorphic VT compared to only 3% of the 31 patients with normal SAECGs. Most of the patients with VT had prior MI and the authors found that the SAECG predicted VT with similar predictive accuracy regardless of whether the MI was anterior or inferior, in contradistinction to the results of Buxton et al.[60] However, both studies are relatively small, making subgroup analysis hazardous.

Recently, the same group performed a similar study in a more homogeneous referred group of 57 patients,[63] all of whom had prior MI and nonsustained VT, although 20 had prior syncope. Clinical variables such as LVEF, left ventricular wall motion, and site of MI did not predict inducible VT (again, the combination of sustained and nonsustained monomorphic VT). The results of SAECG were strongly associated with VT induction, regardless of how the SAECG results were defined. All patients were then treated with antiarrhythmic drugs, guided by EPS in some, or empiric amiodarone or other drugs in others, and were followed-up. The study did not randomly allocate drug treatment or have a control group, but clinical factors within the entire treated and nontreated patient groups were examined with respect to prognosis. The ejection fraction, results of EPS, and adherence to drug therapy were all associated with patient outcome. The SAECG, however, was not tested as a predictor of long-term outcome.

Although the total number of patients studied has not been overwhelming, there is a consistency of results in patients after MI with nonsustained VT; the results of programmed ventricular stimulation can be predicted by the SAECG with good, although imperfect, accuracy. Because about three quarters of these patients will not have inducible VT, there are great advantages to screening out those with a low risk of having a positive EPS result. The SAECG is typically advantageous in this regard due to its high negative predictive accuracy. Effective screening would result in major cost savings by avoiding EPS in a sizable proportion of the total at-risk population. Based on the observations of these published studies, the inducibility rate of VT is approximately 25%; the negative predictive accuracy of the SAECG for this endpoint is approximately 90% (dependent on SAECG definitions). In a hypothetical group of 100 patients with ischemic heart disease and nonsustained VT, one could expect to correctly screen out 54 patients, miss EPS inducibility in only two or three patients, identify EPS inducibility correctly in 22 patients, and perform EPS in 21 noninducible patients. It is unknown whether the EPS or the SAECG provides stronger prognostic data and thus how patients with discordant SAECG and EPS results should be risk-stratified.

The aforementioned approach presupposes that the EPS is the optimal test to predict arrhythmic outcome and that it provides patient-specific data that can be used to guide drug or device therapy. An alternative strategy could be based on a noninvasive approach to maximal risk stratification followed by nonguided therapy such as amiodarone. This method could avoid more costly testing and treatment interventions. Amiodarone is being evaluated in several ongoing treatment trials, although none specifically target patients with MI, left ventricular dysfunction, and nonsustained VT. More long-term data, without contamination by drug therapy, would help clarify the use of the SAECG (or other noninvasive tests, singly and in combination) as a tool to predict patient outcome and its use as a potential noninvasive surrogate or alternative to the EPS.

Prognostic Value of the Signal-Averaged Electrocardiogram in Patients with Idiopathic Dilated Cardiomyopathy or with Advanced Heart Failure

Idiopathic dilated cardiomyopathy is a primary myocardial disease of uncertain etiology that is characterized by left ventricular or biventricular enlargement and impaired contractility. Ventricular arrhythmias are a common manifestation of idiopathic dilated cardiomyopathy. From a review of published studies, it was apparent that 12% of patients with idiopathic dilated cardiomyopathy die suddenly and that 28% of all deaths were sudden.[64] Although it is generally assumed that sudden cardiac death can be equated with fatal VTs, recent analysis[65] of hospitalized patients with severe heart failure suggested nontachyarrhythmic events such as bradyarrhythmias, embolic events, or electromechanical dissociation may actually outnumber sudden deaths due to VT/VF. Clearly, additional insight into the mechanism of sudden death in patients with idiopathic dilated cardiomyopathy, especially in the outpatient setting, will be helpful in understanding, predicting, and ultimately preventing fatal outcomes in these patients.

Patients with idiopathic dilated cardiomyopathy may present with sustained monomorphic VT, polymorphic VT, or VF. The mechanisms involved are more diverse than in coronary heart disease and may include reentry as well as those due to triggered and abnormal automaticity. In addition, such factors as abnormal electrolytes, high circulating levels of catecholamines, myocardial stretch, and decreased myocardial contractility may all play a role in the pathogenesis of ventricular arrhythmias. At least in some patients, particularly those with monomorphic VT, reentry is the likely mechanism. Support for reentry is based on the presence of VT that can be initiated, entrained, and terminated by programmed ventricular stimulation.

Disorders of ventricular conduction on the ECG are common in idiopathic dilated cardiomyopathy. BBB, especially left BBB, is very frequent and correlates with the severity of disease including the degree of interstitial fibrosis. Nonspecific intraventricular conduction defects are also a common ECG finding. Because interstitial fibrosis is a component of the pathology of idiopathic dilated cardiomyopathy, it can cause conduction abnormalities of the specialized conduction system (as seen on the standard ECG), but also disordered ventricular myocardial activation (as seen on SAECG). The extent of myocardial fibrosis as detected by endomyocardial biopsy has correlated with the degree of abnormality of standard SAECG variables.[66]

Clinical, hemodynamic, electrocardiographic, and electrophysiological variables have never demonstrated strong associations with the development of sudden cardiac death in patients with idiopathic dilated cardiomyopathy. The search for useful predictors has continued and a few studies have naturally focused on the SAECG in patients with idiopathic dilated cardiomyopathy. The volume of literature on this subject is a but a fraction of that published about patients with coronary artery disease, despite the scarcity of adequate noninvasive prognostic tools.

A comparison of SAECG results was performed by Poll et al.[67] using patients with idiopathic dilated cardiomyopathy with and without a history of VT/VF. The 29 patients without VTs had a filtered QRSd of 105 ± 13 msec, much less prolonged than the 12 patients with ventricular arrhythmias whose filtered QRSd averaged

130 ± 20 msec. The filtered QRS durations of both groups were significantly longer than normal controls. Importantly, 92% of patients with VT/VF had a QRSd longer than 110 msec versus only 34% in the group without VT/VF. Similar differences were observed for voltage in the terminal 40 msec of the QRS. Patients with BBB were not excluded from this study. The presence of a prolonged filtered QRSd >110 msec and a late potential identified patients with VT/VF with a sensitivity of 83% and a specificity of 86%. Patients with VT/VF could not be distinguished from their counterparts without VT/VF by QRSd on standard ECG or by ejection fraction.

This relatively small study raised the possibility that patients with idiopathic dilated cardiomyopathy prone to VT/VF could be predicted with the SAECG. However, this report was a retrospective analysis undoubtedly influenced by referral bias. Confirmation would be required by prospective evaluation.

In contrast, another study found no difference in time domain measures of the SAECG when patients with VT were compared to patients without VT, all of whom had idiopathic dilated cardiomyopathy.[68] There were trends to greater abnormality on the SAECG in the sustained VT patients relative to the patients with nonsustained VT, but the difference did not reach statistical significance (these subgroups were not compared with the non-VT patients). Frequency domain analyses were also performed. The spectrotemporal mapping results did not correlate with VT; the results of spectral turbulence analysis showed only inconsistent abnormal findings in the VT group. It should be emphasized that a large number of patients were excluded from inclusion in this data set because of chronic antiarrhythmic therapy; thus the remainder of the patients represent a highly selected group. The patients with left BBB were analyzed separately with different normal SAECG values. Therefore, the results of this study did not confirm those of Poll et al.[67] Specifically, the SAECG was more often normal than abnormal even in patients with VT. If confirmed, this low sensitivity for VT (38%) would make the SAECG a poor choice for a screening test in patients with idiopathic dilated cardiomyopathy.

In 1985, the first prospective evaluation of the SAECG was performed in individuals with idiopathic dilated cardiomyopathy.[69] The study was small, enrolling only 42 patients at a single institution. All patients underwent signal averaging, Holter monitoring, and programmed ventricular stimulation, and were followed for 16 months. SAECG analysis was performed in an unusual manner; 12 ECG leads (some internally reconstructed) were visually analyzed after filtering. When low amplitude activity was apparent at least 10 msec after the end of the QRS complex in at least 6 of 12 leads, a late potential was present. Patients with BBB were included and not segregated for analysis. Only 30 patients had an SAECG recorded and in only one patient was the recording abnormal. No patient had monomorphic VT induced with programmed stimulation. Nonsustained VT was common, observed in 38% of Holter recordings. During follow-up, there were only two sudden deaths and there were five deaths due to heart failure.

The small number of sudden deaths in this study preclude any type of predictive analysis of clinical variables. The composite endpoint of sudden and congestive heart failure death was also too small for meaningful interpretation. The most one could conclude from this study was that indicators of an electrical substrate for VT due to reentry (both SAECG and programmed stimulation) were very uncommon in patients with idiopathic dilated cardiomyopathy and thus not likely to be useful as prognostic tools. Clearly, additional study was needed given the conflicting results in this patient population.

More recently, significant progress was made with data from the University of Pennsylvania.[70] These researchers organized a group of 114 patients referred to their center for evaluation of heart failure or for cardiac transplantation; this then represents a highly selected subset of all heart failure patients. Detailed work-up led to the diagnosis of nonischemic cardiomyopathy in all patients, half of whom were termed idiopathic and the other half had a variety of primary causes. Patients without BBB had SAECG recording at baseline. All patients were followed for the development of death, sustained ventricular arrhythmias, or urgent need for cardiac transplantation. Some patients received antiarrhythmic medications and a few had an implantable cardioverter-defibrillator.

Survival curves were generated for the entire cohort divided into three subgroups: patients with a normal SAECG (n=66), patients with an abnormal SAECG (n=20), and patients with BBB (n=28). There were striking differences in event-free survival among these subgroups using several different composite and individual endpoints, but the group with an abnormal SAECG consistently fared worst. For example, survival at 1 year without VT or death was 95% for patients with a normal SAECG, 88% for patients with BBB, but a startling 39% for patients with an abnormal SAECG, as seen in Figure 6.11. This observation was highly statistically significant. In fact, the risk of any endpoint event in the presence

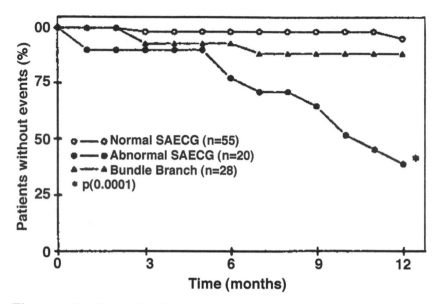

Figure 6.11. Survival with sustained ventricular arrhythmia or death in patients based on presence of normal or abnormal SAECG, or BBB. Patients with abnormal SAECG had a much higher event rate than the other two groups. (Reprinted with permission from Circulation; Mancini et al.[70])

of an abnormal SAECG was increased 17-fold relative to the other subgroups. Additional analyses eliminating patients on antiarrhythmic drugs or patients with a previous history of serious ventricular arrhythmias did not alter the findings. Univariate predictors of adverse outcomes included the SAECG, NYHA classification, peak oxygen consumption, QRSd >120 msec on standard ECG, past history of VT, and gender. With multivariate analysis, only SAECG and NYHA classification predicted the endpoints.

These results strongly support the notion that similar electrophysiological processes may be at work in patients with idiopathic dilated cardiomyopathy and in patients with coronary artery disease. Presumably the presence of myocardial fibrosis resulted in disorganized ventricular conduction and thus abnormalities on SAECG. The SAECG identified a small subset of patients with an alarmingly high rate of fatal or serious events. It appeared that the SAECG results reflected a primary abnormality rather than a measure of disease severity because patients with abnormal SAECG were comparable to patients with normal SAECG in a variety of variables reflecting ventricular performance. One cautionary note regarding this study is that the incidence of sudden death and sustained VT was low, possibly reflecting the benefits of contemporary therapy of heart failure patients. Survival analysis was performed on composite endpoints rather than specific arrhythmic endpoints, and relative risks of individual factors undoubtedly had broad confidence intervals.

However, alone among many variables tested over many years, the SAECG was able to predict VT and death. Moreover, a normal SAECG, a surprisingly common finding, portended an excellent outcome. Whether the SAECG will be an important tool for the selection of specific antiarrhythmic treatment (e.g., amiodarone, implantable defibrillator) will be determined in future clinical trials.

These authors also suggested that the SAECG may represent a promising technique for risk stratification in cardiac transplant candidates, especially given the acute shortage of donor hearts. However, in patients accepted for transplantation, two studies found that no single SAECG variable, or combination, predicted mortality.[71,72]

Patients with severe heart failure are frequently prone to alterations in hemodynamic parameters, especially to fluctuations in ventricular filling pressure. Acute and/or marked changes in ventricular filling pressures could potentially intensify coronary ischemia and adrenergic tone. In addition, the ventricular action potential is sensitive to changes in ventricular filling. Changes in the SAECG during heart failure decompensation would provide mechanistic information and also provide improved guidelines for its use. However, a comprehensive analysis of the SAECG during aggressive therapy of congestive heart failure showed no major changes indicating a stable conduction substrate regardless of hemodynamic status.[73]

Patients with Idiopathic Dilated Cardiomyopathy and Nonsustained Ventricular Tachycardia

Patients with idiopathic dilated cardiomyopathy and nonsustained VT were exclusively reported in a recent publication.[74] In general, these patients have had much lower inducibility rates than comparable patients with ischemic cardiomyopathy, and in this study only 13% of the 70 patients enrolled had inducible sustained monomorphic VT. This study also included patients with syncope; had they been excluded, the inducibility rate would have been only 7%. This and similar previously published results, and our own unpublished observations, lead us to question the clinical value of pursuing EPS in this population when the yield is so low when patients are truly asymptomatic. Nonetheless, the analysis in this study found that only a history of syncope and time-domain SAECG results predicted inducibility. Other factors such as patient age, EF, Holter results, and spectral turbulence analysis of SAECG did not. One of the great disadvantages in patients with idiopathic dilated cardiomyopathy in respect to the SAECG is the high prevalence of intraventricular conduction defects, which may make SAECG analysis unreliable. When these patients were excluded (20 of the 70 in the report), the sensitivity and specificity for sustained VT were excellent, 80% and 96%, respectively. Among all analyzed variables, the SAECG was most strongly associated with EPS results, correctly classifying 86% of patients. Interestingly, the SAECG was abnormal in a relatively small number of the total group of patients (16%), a proportion similar to those with inducible VT, although intraventricular conduction defects-specific normal SAECG values were used.

The use of the SAECG to predict inducible sustained monomorphic VT in patients with idiopathic dilated cardiomyopathy and nonsustained VT will be severely hampered by the low prevalence of electrically induced VT at EPS, a finding that makes EPS use in this patient population controversial. Only one study provides data regarding the results of SAECG and EPS, and long-term prognosis in the specific population of patients with idiopathic dilated cardiomyopathy and nonsustained VT.[75] A series of 80 patients were enrolled; 20 patients had prior syncope and 25 had BBB. The SAECG was abnormal in only 15% of the total group, and sustained monomorphic VT was induced in only 13%, all of whom received chronic amiodarone. Clearly the event rate during follow-up of 22 months could be influenced by the absence of a suitable control group since amiodarone was given uniformly to patients with inducible VT. With these qualifications, survival analysis revealed similar arrhythmia event rates regardless of EPS result and regardless of SAECG result. Given these failures, the authors suggested that more accurate risk stratification modalities were needed to predict sudden death in patients with idiopathic dilated cardiomyopathy.

The absence of a trial involving a large number of asymptomatic idiopathic dilated cardiomyopathy patients with nonsustained VT preferably treated in a controlled and randomized manner (or simply followed without drug treatment) makes it impossible to draw any firm conclusions about the role of SAECG as a prognostic tool. The low inducibility rate at EPS and the concern that sudden death in patients with idiopathic dilated cardiomyopathy is frequently not due to VT[76] further hamper extrapolation of currently available data. At the present time, all that can be concluded is that optimal noninvasive or invasive stratification schemes for patients with idiopathic dilated cardiomyopathy and nonsustained VT are undefined.

Predicting Electrically Induced Ventricular Tachycardia in the Electrophysiology Laboratory in Patients with Unexplained Syncope

Syncope is defined as an episode of transient loss of consciousness due to cerebral hypoperfusion. The causes of syncope are many but can be reasonably characterized as cardiac and noncardiac (such as neurological or metabolic). Further categorization as a cardiac cause typically breaks down as mechanical, arrhythmic, and reflex diagnoses.

More than one third of all people will have at least one syncopal event in their lifetime. Most events are benign, nonrecurrent, and do not require extensive evaluation or treatment. Syncope is a common reason for evaluation in the emergency room setting, and it also accounts for many hospital admissions and referrals for further diagnostic investigations. Many patients will have the cause of syncope identified on initial examination and not require additional testing beyond routine examination and blood work. However, in some patients the mechanism of syncope is elusive and requires provocative testing; this situation is commonly termed unexplained syncope and implies that a diagnosis is not easily or readily attained without special investigation.

The classification of syncope into cardiac and noncardiac causes is important for guiding work-up and also for prognosis. Whereas noncardiac syncope has a mortality rate as low as 0%, cardiac syncope has been reported to carry a 1-year incidence of sudden death as high as 24%.[77] In order to clarify the mechanism of syncope when it remains unexplained, patients are frequently referred for further testing. The EPS is used to provide information supportive of a variety of bradyarrhythmic and tachyarrhythmic cardiac diagnoses, and provides relevant information in at least half of the cases. In anywhere from 15% to 35% of cases, sustained VT is diagnosed as the cause of syncope. This diagnosis is particularly important because undiagnosed syncopal VT may recur and may be fatal. Untreated

VT carries a substantial risk and successful suppression reduces the risk of VT recurrence and sudden death.

Many patients with unexplained syncope have a nondiagnostic EPS procedure and may require other forms of provocative testing (such as tilt table study). EPS is also invasive and not universally available. For these reasons, several efforts have been mounted to predict which patients are more likely to have a diagnostic EPS and in particular which patients are most likely to have the most serious of arrhythmic diagnoses, sustained VT.

In a small study of 24 patients with syncope, SAECG was performed prior to EPS.[78] Sustained VT was diagnosed in nine patients. The filtered QRS duration was strikingly different in the patients with VT (152 ± 25 msec) in contrast to the patients who had no VT (113 ± 8 msec). There was nearly complete separation of induced VT patients from those without induced VT based on the QRSd on SAECG. The authors reasoned that the SAECG may be useful to screen for high-risk patients who require programmed ventricular stimulation.

A much larger prospective study also highlighted the SAECG. A variety of diagnoses were found by prolonged ECG monitoring and by EPS in 150 patients. EPS was performed only in a select subset, and VT was diagnosed in 22 subjects but was sustained in only 12 (spontaneous VT in four and induced VT in eight). For the diagnosis of VT, the SAECG had a sensitivity of 73%, a specificity of 89%, and a predictive accuracy of 54%. These investigators also highlighted the importance of the combination of heart disease and the SAECG; the presence of coronary artery disease and an abnormal SAECG had a predictive accuracy of 82%.

Holter ECG recording is almost always performed as part of the work-up for the syncopal patient. Winters et al.[79] examined both the SAECG as well as the quantity of ventricular arrhythmias on the Holter recordings in 40 patients with undiagnosed syncope. Neither the frequency of ventricular premature beats nor the presence of nonsustained VT was related to the presence of inducible VT. In contradistinction, the SAECG-derived variables distinguished patients with inducible VT from those without VT. The sensitivity of individual SAECG variables ranged between 50% and 83% and the specificity ranged between 82% and 91%, with the strongest association between VT and the V40 results.

Another study[80] compared SAECG with body surface potential mapping as markers for risk of VT induced in the EP laboratory. Body surface mapping is infrequently used for clinical purposes but can provide unique descriptions of the geographic distribution of areas of abnormal repolarization across the surface of the thoracic cavity. In this study, this technique failed to identify those patients who had inducible VT, whereas the SAECG was useful.

These small studies suggested that the SAECG may be useful as a screening test for VT in patients who have unexplained syncope, but interpretation was hampered by several design flaws such as small sample size, use of spontaneous nonsustained VT as an endpoint, and failure to perform programmed stimulation with three extrastimuli to maximize sensitivity of EPS. Although some comparisons were made with other potentially useful noninvasive screening tests, these studies lacked sufficient power to perform meaningful comparisons. Finally, the presence and severity of underlying structural heart disease was not controlled in the statistical analyses.

Most recently, a multicenter group of investigators collected prospective data on a large number of patients with at least one episode of unexplained syncope or severe near-syncope who were referred to the respective institutions.[52] There were 189 patients enrolled, of whom about one quarter had either prior MI or nonischemic left ventricular dysfunction and about one third had no identifiable heart disease. Sustained monomorphic VT was induced in 28 patients or 15% of the total group; a detailed analysis of potential predictors of inducible VT was undertaken.

Patients with VT were neither older nor characterized by gender. However, one piece of historical data was different: more than three times as many patients with VT had a history of prior MI as patients without VT (Table 6.4). As previously suggested, the results of Holter recording had no correlation with VT inducibility.

All SAECG variables were associated with VT as shown in Table 6.5, although the most striking differences was observed with the fQRS determination. Of the group with VT, 70% had a fQRS prolonged >110 msec compared to only 45% of those without VT (p= 0.02).

As has been emphasized throughout the text, the SAECG can be defined clinically in a variety of ways, a process that will affect the predictive value of the abnormal test. The SAECG typically generates three measurements or calculations: fQRS, V40, and low-amplitude signal. Several normal values of fQRS have appeared in the literature, whereas V40 and LAS have generally had only single normal value used. Whether these SAECG component measurements have been used in combination or alone varies throughout the published SAECG experience. This large syncope study provided

Table 6.4

Characteristics of Patients with (Group 1) and Without (Group 2)
Inducible Ventricular Tachycardia

	Group 1 (n = 28)	Group 2 (n = 156)	p Value
Age (yr)	61 ± 14	58 ± 16	NS
Male	20 (74)	98 (61)	NS
Previous MI	11 (39)	19 (12)	<0.001
EF	0.40 ± 0.16	0.50 ± 0.16	0.02
<0.40	10/18 (56)	21/83 (25)	0.02
Abnormal Holter recording	15/21 (71)	46/79 (51)	NS
≥10 VPDs/hour on Holter recording	13/19 (68)	38/71 (54)	NS
≥1 Run NSVT on Holter recording	10/16 (63)	23/56 (41)	NS

Values presented are mean value ± SD or number (%) of patients. EF = ejection fraction; MI = myocardial infarction; NSVT = nonsustained ventricular tachycardia; VPDs = ventricular premature depolarizations. (Adapted from JACC; Steinberg JS, et al.[52])

Table 6.5

Results of Signal-Averaged Electrocardiogram in Patients with
(Group 1) and without (Group 2) Inducible Ventricular Tachycardia

	Group 1 (n = 28)	Group 2 (n = 156)	p Value
fQRS (msec)	120 ± 24	105 ± 17	<0.005
>110 msec	18 (67)	48 (31)	<0.001
>114 msec	16 (57)	41 (25)	<0.005
>120 msec	10 (36)	24 (15)	<0.02
V40 (μV)	28 ± 30	37 ± 28	NS
>20 μV	14 (50)	49 (31)	0.05
LAS (msec)	43 ± 23	34 ± 13	<0.01
>38 msec	14 (50)	46 (29)	0.03

Values presented are mean value ± SD or number (%) of patients. fQRS = filtered QRS vector magnitude; LAS = low-amplitude signal duration; V40 = root mean square voltage of the terminal 40 msec of the vector complex. (Adapted from JACC; Steinberg JS, et al.[52])

an opportunity to examine various definitions of SAECG and the relationship with a valid clinical endpoint. As one can discern from Figure 6.12, as the fQRS cutpoint was lengthened, sensitivity measurably declined and specificity improved. More demonstrable changes were made by requiring two or three variables abnormal.

In a similar fashion, using the SAECG with clinical variables will affect the predictive value. In Figure 6.13, a receiver operator curve was constructed using three variables (prior MI, EF <0.40,

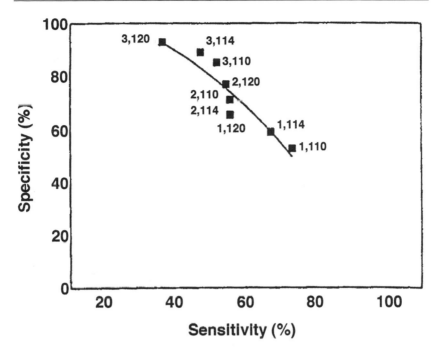

Figure 6.12. Receiver operator curve for results of the SAECG predicting inducible VT at electrophysiological study. The SAECG results were defined by the number of criteria (1, 2, or 3) required for a positive result and the filtered QRS duration cutpoint (110, 114, or 120 msec). (Reprinted with permission from JACC; Steinberg et al.[52])

and SAECG) alone and in various combinations. The SAECG had the highest sensitivity but poor specificity. Although history of prior MI or a low ejection fraction was a more specific finding, the sensitivity of each was low. Combining variables improved sensitivity, specificity, or both. The combination of prior MI and abnormal SAECG had an excellent specificity. In addition, this combination yielded a high positive predictive value: 60% of these patients had inducible VT. The absence of history of MI, low ejection fraction, or SAECG abnormality had excellent sensitivity and a low risk of VT (negative predictive value of 93%).

With multivariate analysis, only two variables were identified as independent: a history of prior MI and the SAECG results. The risk of inducible VT was increased several-fold if either or both was present as shown graphically in Figure 6.14. The SAECG thus identified a unique feature of the patients'clinical profile: myocardial conduction delay in the absence of BBB.

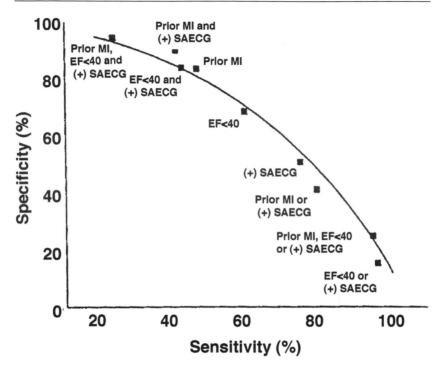

Figure 6.13. Receiver operator curve for single and recombination clinical variables. EF <40 = ejection fraction <0.40, MI = myocardial infarction. (Reprinted with permission from JACC; Steinberg et al.[52])

Using logistic regression techniques, a model was created based on the use of sequential performed tests in order to determine the incremental predictive value of noninvasive screening for inducible VT in patients with unexplained syncope. Based on history, in essence the presence of prior MI, two groups were formed: a low-risk group with a probability range for VT of 5% to 13% and a moderate-risk group with a probability range for VT of 28% to 42%. History alone could not assign risk above 50%.

The SAECG, when added to the history model, added significant incremental information to the total group. Interestingly, the SAECG had no incremental predictive value for the low-risk group. Thus, the presence of an abnormal SAECG when no history of MI exists meant it was likely a false positive result. Of the moderate-risk group (history of MI), the SAECG was able to stratify risk—the risk was twice as high when the SAECG was abnormal. Thus, the SAECG performed well with these "gray zone" patients.

Odds Ratio for Inducible
Ventricular Tachycardia

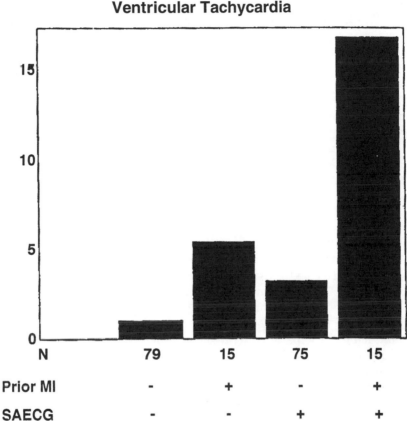

Figure 6.14. In a study of 189 patients, two variables (history of prior myocardial infarction [MI] and positive findings on the SAECG) were independently predictive of inducible VT in patients with syncope. The relative risk of inducible VT of individual and combination variables is indicated. (Reprinted with permission from JACC; Steinberg et al.[52])

Adding the ejection fraction as the second variable (after history and before other tests), yielded results similar to those for SAECG, but was less predictive. Holter results as the second test were only of borderline significance.

When adding tests third in a sequence, none was able to increment predictive value. For example, the SAECG could not meaningfully improve prediction if history and ejection fraction were already known. The SAECG or any noninvasive test was not powerful enough to impart significant prognostic information when used later in the sequence of screening.

The low-risk group presented a particular screening problem because it represented about 80% of the patients. Only the combination of an abnormal SAECG using the most stringent definition (fQRS >120 msec and all three criteria abnormal) and a Holter revealing frequent or complex ventricular arrhythmia significantly predicted greater risk of inducible VT. Patients without prior MI may be particularly problematic because of problems inherent in the screening tests or in the EPS itself.

This study therefore confirmed the high sensitivity of the SAECG for VT in this patient population, but also emphasized its high false positive rate, an observation not made previously. The SAECG thus performs best to exclude risk rather than to identify high risk. However, different definitions of the SAECG or use of SAECG in combination with other clinical variables largely attenuates this deficiency of the SAECG. The use of the SAECG can be customized to the needs of the user. In clinical practice, screening with a sensitive test is usually desired given the needs of the individual patient. Clinical trials might select a highly specific approach if intervention or treatment has risk.

Clearly, the SAECG has a prominent role to play as a predictor of inducible VT in patients with unexplained syncope. The laboratory induction of VT has important implications for treatment. Further prospective study will be needed to answer whether the SAECG predicts VT or sudden death in these patients.

Use of the Signal-Averaged Electrocardiogram in Other Forms of Heart Disease

Signal-averaged electrocardiography has been applied to a number of other forms of heart disease and clinical entities that are less common or have a lower prevalence of VTs than those reviewed in the preceding sections. The published experience in these patient populations is formative and at present, use of the SAECG for many of these indications must be considered investigational. This section will briefly describe some of the data available in this subject area.

When patients experience VT yet have structurally normal hearts after extensive evaluation, they are said to have idiopathic VT. Most idiopathic VT originates in the right ventricular outflow tract and to a lesser extent the posteroseptal left ventricle. One study[81] of 40 patients with idiopathic VT found that the SAECG was more abnormal in these patients than in normal subjects but less abnormal than in patients with ischemic heart disease. The incidence of late potentials was also intermediate: 0% in normal subjects, 20% in idiopathic VT (37% in those with sustained VT), and 58% in VT related to ischemic heart disease. Interestingly, the presence of abnormal myocardial histology was strongly related to the presence of late potentials, suggesting that conduction delay was indeed related to fibrosis even in the absence of gross structural abnormality. The lower incidence of SAECG abnormality in idiopathic VT probably relates to the greater diversity of mechanisms responsible for VT, the lesser degree of conduction delay observed even if reentry is present, and the smaller myocardial mass that generates conduction delay. In our experience, the SAECG is usually normal in patients with idiopathic VT, and the SAECG has little role in the clinical management of these patients.

Arrhythmogenic right ventricular dysplasia is a rare syndrome characterized by replacement of myocardial tissue with adipose tissue, right ventricular cardiomyopathy, and recurrent left BBB VT due to reentry. In the largest description of the SAECG in arrhythmogenic right ventricular dysplasia, Kinoshita et al.[82] examined 28 patients with arrhythmogenic right ventricular dysplasia and VT and 35 normal subjects. In this disorder, it is unfortunately rarely possible to study patients with pathological arrhythmogenic right ventricular dysplasia but no clinical expression of VT. Relative to controls, patients with arrhythmogenic right ventricular dysplasia had much greater fQRS prolongation at 25 Hz and 40 Hz filter settings; patients' fQRS exceeded controls by approximately 25 msec. Late potentials were present in about two thirds of arrhythmogenic right ventricular dysplasia patients but not in any of the controls. Sensitivity of the time domain SAECG was enhanced by combination with frequency domain SAECG results; the authors suggested that this combination may be useful as a screening test for arrhythmogenic right ventricular dysplasia. In our experience, some of the most abnormal SAECG tracings may be recorded in arrhythmogenic right ventricular dysplasia patients. It can by used clinically to indicate the underlying anatomic substrate in patients with left BBB VT whose heart disease is undiagnosed or who have minimal findings during preliminary work-up, which stands in contradistinction to patients with idiopathic VT.

Sudden cardiac death may sometimes occur in patients with hypertrophic cardiomyopathy. It is postulated that VTs may be a major cause of sudden death in this population, and identification of those at greatest risk is of intense intrinsic interest. This is particularly important in that hypertrophic cardiomyopathy is a major cause of unexpected or sudden death in young patients. The largest study looking at an array of noninvasive data to predict sudden death in hypertrophic cardiomyopathy was performed by Cripps et al.[83] in 1990. Sixty-four patients were examined at a referral center. An abnormal SAECG was detected in 20% of the patients with hypertrophic cardiomyopathy, but in only 4% of a group of 50 normal subjects. SAECG was not correlated with important clinical parameters such as family history of sudden death, a history of syncope, or the degree of left ventricular hypertrophy on echocardiography. Of the patients with nonsustained VT on Holter monitoring, a previously described risk factor for sudden death, approximately half had an abnormal SAECG. Unfortunately, this was not a prospective study so it is impossible to be certain whether the SAECG can accurately predict those who will experience sudden death in this population. This study was also limited by the fact that a substantial number of patients were on chronic amiodarone, which may create abnormalities on the SAECG that would not have been present in the absence of antiarrhythmic drug treatment. In the young patients with hypertrophic cardiomyopathy, there is pressure to develop risk stratification schema for sudden death; unfortunately, the number of patients of a young age in this study with clinical significant arrhythmias was too small for meaningful analysis. Because an SAECG seems to detect a unique electrical abnormality not strongly related to myocardial or hemodynamic measurements, further investigation of the SAECG and its potential role for predicting either spontaneous arrhythmic events or electrically induced ventricular arrhythmias is clearly indicated.

Patients with surgically repaired tetralogy of Fallot may rarely develop late postoperative VT or sudden death. Because of the ubiquitous presence of right BBB after surgical repair, adjustment of SAECG criteria must be made. The SAECG has been reported to correlate with the inducibility of VT by programmed stimulation.[84] In patients with mitral valve prolapse, the SAECG may be abnormal in a substantial minority,[85] but correlation with sustained VTs is lacking. In myotonic dystrophy, cardiac arrhythmias may develop and sudden death is not uncommon. The SAECG is abnormal in many of these patients and these observations suggest that VTs due to reentry may be responsible for some of the observed instances of sudden death.[86]

References

1. Simson MB. Use of signals in the terminal QRS complex to identify patients with ventricular tachycardia after myocardial infarction. Circulation 64:235-242, 1981.
2. Breithardt G, Borggrefe M, Karbenn U, Abendroth RR, Yeh HL, Seipel L. Prevalence of late potentials in patients with and without ventricular tachycardia: Correlation with angiographic findings. Am J Cardiol 49;1932-1937, 1982.
3. Gomes AJ, Winters S, Martinson M, Machac J, Stewart D, Targonski A. The prognostic significance of quantitative signal-averaged variables relative to clinical variables, site of myocardial infarction, ejection fraction and ventricular premature beats: A prospective study. J Am Coll Cardiol 13:377-384, 1989.
4. Steinberg JS, Regan A, Sciacca RR, Bigger JT, Fleiss JL, Salvatore DE, Fosina M, Rolnitsky LM. Predicting arrhythmic events after acute myocardial infarction using the signal-averaged electrocardiogram. Am J Cardiol 69:13-21, 1992.
5. Breithardt G, Borggrefe M, Quantius B, Karbenn U, Seipel L. Ventricular vulnerability assessed by programmed ventricular stimulation in patients with and without late potentials. Circulation 68:275-281, 1983.
6. Richards DA, Blake GJ, Spear JF, Moore EN. Electrophysiologic substrate for ventricular tachycardia: Correlation of properties in vivo and in vitro. Circulation 69:369-381, 1984.
7. Borbola J, Ezri MD, Denes P. Correlation between the signal-averaged electrocardiogram and electrophysiologic study findings in patients with coronary artery disease and sustained ventricular tachycardia. Am Heart J 115:816-824, 1988.
8. Freedman RA, Gillis AM, Keren A, Sodorholm-Difatte V, Mason J. Signal-averaged electrocardiographic late potentials in patients with ventricular fibrillation or ventricular tachycardia: Correlation with clinical arrhythmia and electrophysiologic study. Am J Cardiol 55:1350-1353, 1985.
9. Agarwal JB, Naccarrella FF, Weintraub WS, Helfant RH. Sinus rhythm mapping in healed experimental myocardial infarction: Contrasting activation patterns for inducing ventricular tachycardia versus fibrillation. Am J Cardiol 55:1601-1607, 1985.
10. Steinberg JS, Smith R, Bigger JT, Jr, Damm CJ. Determinants of the signal averaged ECG after myocardial infarction: Relationship to infarct size and site in an experimental canine model. PACE 12:665, 1989.
11. El-Sherif N, Scherlag BJ, Lazzara R. Electrode catheter recordings during malignant ventricular arrhythmia following experimental acute myocardial ischemia. Circulation 51:1003-1014, 1975.
12. Gardner PI, Ursell PC, Pham TD, Fenoglio JJ, Wit AL. Electrophysiologic and anatomic basis for fractionated electrograms recorded from healed myocardial infarcts. Circulation 72:596-611, 1984.

13. Fenoglio JJ, Pham TD, Harken AH, Horowitz LN, Josephson ME, Wit AL. Recurrent sustained ventricular tachycardia: Structure and ultrastructure of subendocardial regions in which tachycardia originates. Circulation 68:518-533, 1983.
14. McGuire M, Kuchar D, Ganis J, Sammel N, Thorburn C. Natural history of late potentials in the first ten days after acute myocardial infarction and relation to early ventricular arrhythmias. Am J Cardiol 62:1197-1190, 1988.
15. Kertes PJ, Glabus M, Murray A, Julian DG, Campbell RWF. Delayed ventricular depolarization: Correlation with ventricular activation and relevance to ventricular fibrillation in acute myocardial infarction. Eur Heart J 5:974-983, 1984.
16. Gomes AJ, Mehra R, Barreca P, El-Sherif N, Hariman R, Holtzman R. Quantitative analysis of the high frequency components of the signal-averaged QRS complex in patients with acute myocardial infarction: A prospective study. Circulation 72:105-111, 1985.
17. Hong M, Peter T, Peters W, Wang FZ, Xiu Y, Vaughn C, Gang ES. Relation between acute ventricular arrhythmias, ventricular late potentials and mortality in acute myocardial infarction. Am J Cardiol 68:1403-1409, 1991.
18. Janse MJ, Kléber AJ. Electrophysiological changes and ventricular arrhythmias in the early phase of regional myocardial infarction. Circ Res 49:1069-1081, 1981.
19. Breithardt G, Schwarzmaier J, Borggrefe M, Haerten K, Seipel L. Prognostic significance of late ventricular potentials after acute myocardial infarction. Eur Heart J 4:487-495, 1983.
20. Kuchar DL, Thorburn CW, Sammel N. Late potentials detected after myocardial infarction: Natural history and prognostic significance. Circulation 74:1280-1289, 1986.
21. Denniss AR, Richards DA, Cody DV, Russell PA, Young AA, Cooper MJ, Ross DL, Uther JB. Prognostic significance of ventricular tachycardia and fibrillation induced at programmed stimulation and delayed potentials detected on the signal-averaged electrocardiograms of survivors of acute myocardial infarction. Circulation 74:731-745, 1986.
22. Steinberg JS, Freedman RA, Bigger JT, Jr, and the ESVEM Investigators. Antiarrhythmic drug therapy and the signal-averaged electrocardiogram. In: El-Sherif N, Turitto G (eds). High Resolution Electrocardiography, Futura Publishing Co., Mt. Kisco, NY, pp 569-590, 1992.
23. Kuchar DL, Thorburn CW, Sammel NL. Prediction of serious arrhythmic events after myocardial infarction: Signal-averaged electrocardiogram, Holter monitoring and radionuclide ventriculography. J Am Coll Cardiol 9:531-538, 1987.
24. Denniss AR, Richards DA, Waywood JA, Yung T, Kam CA, Ross DL, Uther JB. Electrophysiological and anatomic differences between canine hearts with inducible ventricular tachycardia and fibrillation associated with chronic myocardial infarction. Circ Res 64:155-166, 1989.
25. Gomes AJ, Winters SL, Stewart D, Horowitz S, Milner M, Barreca P. A new noninvasive index to predict sustained ventricular tachycardia and sudden death in the first year after myocardial infarction: Based

on signal-averaged electrocardiogram, radionuclide ejection fraction and Holter monitoring. J Am Coll Cardiol 10:349-357, 1987.

26. Cripps TR, Bennett ED, Camm AJ, Ward DE. High gain signal averaged electrocardiogram combined with 24-hour monitoring in patients early after myocardial infarction for bedside prediction of arrhythmic events. Br Heart J 60:181-187, 1988.

27. Steinberg JS, Regen A, Sciacca RR, Bigger JT, Fleiss JL. Predicting arrhythmic events after acute myocardial infarction using the signal-averaged electrocardiogram. Am J Cardiol 69:13-21, 1992.

28. El-Sherif N, Denes P, Katz R, Capone R, Mitchell B, Carlson M, Reynolds-Haertle R. Definition of the best prediction criteria of the time domain signal-averaged electrocardiogram for serious arrhythmic events in the postinfarction period. J Am Coll Cardiol 25:908-914, 1995.

29. Farrell TG, Bashir Y, Cripps T, Malik M, Poloniecki J, Bennett ED, Ward DE, Camm AJ. Risk stratification for arrhythmic events in post infarction patients based on heart rate variability, ambulatory electrocardiographic variables and the signal-averaged electrocardiogram. J Am Coll Cardiol 18:687-697, 1991.

30. Odemyuiwa O, Malik M, Poloniecki J, Farrell T, Millane T, Kulakowski P, Staunton A, Matthies A, Camm AJ. Differences between predictive characteristics of signal-averaged electrocardiographic variables for postinfarction sudden death ventricular tachycardia. Am J Cardiol 69:1186-1192, 1992.

31. Vaitkus PT, Kendwall E, Marchlinski FE, Miller JM, Buxton AE, Josephson ME. Differences in electrophysiological substrate in patients with coronary artery disease and cardiac arrest or ventricular tachycardia: Insights from endocardial mapping and signal-averaged electrocardiography. Circulation 84:672-678, 1991.

32. Breithardt G, Borggrefe M, Haerten K. Role of programmed ventricular stimulation and noninvasive recording of ventricular late potentials for the identification of patients at risk of ventricular tachyarrhythmias after acute myocardial infarction. In: Zipes DP, Jalife J (eds). Cardiac Electrophysiology and Arrhythmias, pp 553-561, 1983.

33. Richards D, Byth K, Ross DL, Uther JB. What is the best predictor of spontaneous ventricular tachycardia and sudden death after myocardial infarction? Circulation 83:756-763, 1991.

34. Pedretti R, Etro MD, Laporta A, Braga SS, Carù B. Prediction of late arrhythmic events after acute myocardial infarction from combined use of noninvasive prognostic variables and inducibility of sustained monomorphic ventricular tachycardia. Am J Cardiol 71:1131-1141, 1993.

35. Gang ES, Lew AS, Hong M, Wang FZ, Siebert CA, Peter T. Decreased incidence of ventricular late potentials after successful thrombolytic therapy for acute myocardial infarction. N Engl J Med 321:712-716, 1989.

36. Vatterott PJ, Hammill SC, Bailey KR, Wiltgen CM, Gersh BJ. Late potentials on signal-averaged electrocardiograms and patency of the infarct-related artery in survivors of acute myocardial infarction. J Am Coll Cardiol 17:330-337, 1991.

37. Zimmerman M, Adamec R, Ciaroni S, Malbois F, Tieche R. Reduction in the frequency of ventricular late potentials after acute myocardial infarction by early thrombolytic therapy. Am J Cardiol 67:697-703, 1991.

38. Pedretti R, Laporta A, Etro MD, Gementi A, Bonelli R, Anzà C, Colombo E, Maslowsky F, Santoro F, Carn B. Influence of thrombolysis on signal-averaged electrocardiogram and late arrhythmic events after acute myocardial infarction. Am J Cardiol 69:866-872, 1992.

39. Aguirre FV, Kern MJ, Hsia J, Serota H, Janosik D, Greenwalt T, Ross AM, Chaitman BR. Importance of myocardial infarct artery patency on the prevalence of ventricular arrhythmia and late potentials after thrombolysis in acute myocardial infarction. Am J Cardiol 68:1410-1416, 1991.

40. Lange RA, Cigarroa RG, Wells PJ, Kremers MS, Hillis LD. Influence of anterograde flow in the infarct artery on the incidence of late potentials after acute myocardial infarction. Am J Cardiol 65:554-558, 1990.

41. DeChillou C, Rodriguez L-M, Doevendans P, Loutsidis K, Van den Dool A, Metzger J, Bär F, Smeets J, Wellens H. Factors influencing changes in the signal-averaged electrocardiogram within the first year after a first myocardial infarction. Am Heart J 128:263-270, 1994.

42. Tranchesi B, Verstraete M, Van de Werf F, De Albuquerque CP, Caramelli B, Gebara OC, Pereira WI, Moffa P, Bellotti G, Pileggi F. Usefulness of high-frequency analysis of signal-averaged surface electrocardiograms in acute myocardial infarction before and after coronary thrombolysis for assessing coronary reperfusion. Am J Cardiol 66:1196-1198, 1990.

43. Steinberg JS, Hochman JS, Morgan CD, Dorian P, Naylor CD, Theroux P, Topol EJ, Armstrong PW, and the LATE Ancillary Study Investigators. The effects of thrombolytic therapy administered 6-24 hours after myocardial infarction on the signal-averaged electrocardiogram: Results of a multicenter randomized trial. Circulation 90:746-752, 1994.

44. Boehrer JD, Glamann B, Lange RA, Willard JE, Brogan WC, Eichhorn EJ, Grayburn PA, Anwar A, Hillis LD. Effect of coronary angioplasty on late potentials one to two weeks after acute myocardial infarction. Am J Cardiol 70:1515-1519, 1992.

45. Ragosta M, Sabia PJ, Kaul S, DiMarco J, Sarembock IJ, Powers ER. Effects of late (1 to 30 days) reperfusion after acute myocardial infarction on the signal-averaged electrocardiogram. Am J Cardiol 71:19-23, 1993.

46. Zaman AG, Morris JL, Smyllie JH, Cowan JC. Late potentials and ventricular enlargement after myocardial infarction. Circulation 88:905-914, 1993.

47. Sager PT, Perlmutter RA, Rosenfeld LE, McPherson CA, Wackers FJ, Batsford WP. Electrophysiologic effects of thrombolytic therapy in patients with transmural anterior myocardial infarction complicated by left ventricular aneurysm formation. J Am Coll Cardiol 12:19-24, 1988.

48. Malik M, Kulakowski P, Odemuyiwa O, Poloniecki J, Staunton A, Milane T, Farrell T, Camm AJ. Effect of thrombolytic therapy in the predictive value of signal-averaged electrocardiography after acute myocardial infarction. Am J Cardiol 70:21-25, 1992.

49. McClements BM, Adgey AA. Value of signal-averaged electrocardiography, radionuclide ventriculography, Holter monitoring and clinical variables for prediction of arrhythmic events in survivors of acute myocardial infarction in the thrombolytic era. J Am Coll Cardiol 21:1419-1427, 1993.

50. Denes P, El-Sherif N, Katz R, Capone R, Carlson M, Mitchell B, Ledingham R for the Cardiac Arrhythmia Suppression Trial (CAST) SAECG substudy investigators. Prognostic significance of signal-averaged electrocardiogram after thrombolytic therapy and/or angioplasty during acute myocardial infarction (CAST Substudy). Am J Cardiol 74:216-220, 1994.

51. Hohnloser SH, Franck P, Klingenheben T, Zabel M, Just H. Open infarct artery, late potentials, and other prognostic factors in patients after acute myocardial infarction in the thrombolytic era: A prospective trial. Circulation 90:1747-1756, 1994.

52. Steinberg JS, Prystowsky E, Freedman RA, Moreno F, Katz R, Kron J, Regan A, Sciacca RR. Use of the signal-averaged electrocardiogram for predicting inducible ventricular tachycardia in patients with unexplained syncope: Relation to clinical variables in multivariate analysis. J Am Coll Cardiol 23:99-106, 1994.

53. Verzoni A, Romano S, Pozzoni L, Tarricone D, Sangiorgio S, Croce L. Prognostic significance and evolution of late ventricular potentials in the first year after myocardial infarction: A prospective study. PACE 12:41-51, 1989.

54. Kuchar DL, Thorburn CW, Sammel N. Prognostic implications of loss of late potentials following acute myocardial infarction. PACE 16:2104-2111, 1993.

55. El-Sherif N, Ursell S, Bekheit S, Fontaine J, Turitto G, Henkin R, Caref EB. Prognostic significance of signal-averaged ECG depends on the time of recording in the postinfarction period. Am Heart J 118:256-264, 1989.

56. Rodriguez LM, Krijne R, Van den Dool A, Brugada P, Smeets J, Wellens H. Time course and prognostic significance of serial signal-averaged electrocardiograms after a first acute myocardial infarction. Am J Cardiol 66:1199-1202, 1990.

57. Steinberg JS, Bigger JT, Jr, Damm CJ. Predictors of ventricular tachycardia after experimental myocardial infarction: Use of the signal averaged ECG and infarct size. Circulation 80:II-36, 1989.

58. Kuchar DL, Rosenbaum DS, Ruskin J, Garan H. Late potentials in the signal-averaged electrocardiogram after canine myocardial infarction: Correlation with induced ventricular arrhythmias during the healing phase. JACC 15:1365-1373, 1990.

59. Wilber DJ, Olshansky B, Moran JF, Scanlon PJ. Electrophysiologic testing and nonsustained ventricular tachycardia: Use and limitations in patients with coronary artery disease and impaired ventricular function. Circulation 82:350-358, 1990.

60. Buxton AE, Simson MB, Falcone RA, Marchlinski FE, Doherty JU, Josephson ME. Results of signal-averaged electrocardiography and electrophysiologic study in patients with nonsustained ventricular tachycardia after healing of acute myocardial infarction. Am J Cardiol 60:80-85, 1987.

61. Turitto G, Fontane JM, Ursell SN, Caref EB, Henkin R, El-Sherif N. Value of signal-averaged electrocardiogram as a predictor of the results of programmed stimulation in nonsustained ventricular tachycardia. Am J Cardiol 61:1272-1278, 1988.

62. Winters SL, Stewart D, Targonski A, Gomes AJ. Role of signal-averaging of the surface QRS complex in selecting patients with nonsustained ventricular tachycardia and high grade ventricular arrhythmias for programmed ventricular stimulation. J Am Coll Cardiol 12:1481-1487, 1988.

63. Winters SL, Ip J. Deshmukh P, DeLuca A, Daniels K, Pe E, Gomes JA. Determinants of induction of ventricular tachycardia in nonsustained ventricular tachycardia after myocardial infarction and the usefulness of signal-averaged electrocardiogram. Am J Cardiol 72:1281-1285, 1993.

64. Dec GW, Fuster V. Idiopathic dilated cardiomyopathy. N Engl J Med 331:1564-1575, 1994.

65. Luu M, Stevenson WG, Stevenson LW, Baron K, Walden J. Diverse mechanisms of unexpected cardiac arrest in advanced heart failure. Circulation 80:1675-1680, 1989.

66. Yamada T, Fukunami M, Ohmori M, Iwakura K, Kumagai K, Kondoh N, Tsujimura E, Abe Y, Nagareda T, Kotoh K, Hoki N. New approach to the estimation of the extent of myocardial fibrosis in patients with dilated cardiomyopathy: Use of signal-averaged electrocardiography. Am Heart J 126:626-631, 1993.

67. Poll DS, Marchlinski FE, Falcone MS, Josephson ME, Simson MB. Abnormal signal-averaged electrocardiograms in patients with nonischemic congestive cardiomyopathy: Relationship to sustained ventricular tachyarrhythmias. Circulation 72:1308-1313, 1985.

68. Keeling PJ, Kulakowski P, Yi G, Slade A, Bent SE, McKenna WJ. Usefulness of signal-averaged electrocardiogram in idiopathic dilated cardiomyopathy for identifying patients with ventricular arrhythmias. Am J Cardiol 72:78-84, 1993.

69. Meinertz T, Treese N, Kasper W, Geibel A, Hofmann T, Zehender M, Bohn D, Pop T, Just H. Determinants of prognosis in idiopathic dilated cardiomyopathy as determined by programmed electrical stimulation. Am J Cardiol 56:337-341, 1985.

70. Mancini D, Wong KL, Simson MB. Prognostic value of abnormal signal-averaged electrocardiogram in patients with nonischemic congestive cardiomyopathy. Circulation 87:1083-1092, 1993.

71. Pinsky DJ, Sciacca RR, Steinberg JS. QT dispersion as a marker of risk in patients awaiting heart transplantation. J Am Coll Cardiol 29:1576-1584, 1997.

72. Middlekauff HR, Stevenson WG, Woo MA, Moser DK, Stevenson LW. Comparison of frequency of late potentials in idiopathic dilated cardiomyopathy and ischemic cardiomyopathy with advanced congestive heart failure and their usefulness in predicting sudden death. Am J Cardiol 66:1113-1117, 1990.

73. Stevenson WG, Woo MA, Mosner DK, Stevenson LW. Late potentials are unaltered by ventricular filling pressure reduction in heart failure. Am Heart J 122:473-477, 1991.

74. Turitto G, Ahuja R, Bekheit S, Caref EB, Ibrahim B, El-Sherif N. Incidence and prediction of induced ventricular tachyarrhythmias in idiopathic dilated cardiomyopathy. Am J Cardiol 73:770-773, 1994.

75. Turitto G, Ahuja RK, Caref EB, El-Sherif N. Risk stratification for arrhythmic events in patients with nonischemic dilated cardiomyopathy

and nonsustained ventricular tachycardia: Role of programmed ventricular stimulation and the signal-averaged electrocardiogram. J Am Coll Cardiol 24:1523-1528, 1994.

76. Stevenson WG, Nademanee K, Weiss JN, Weiner I, Baron K, Yeatman LA, Sherman CT. Programmed electrical stimulation at potential ventricular reentry circuit sites: Comparison of observations in humans with predictions from computer simulations. Circulation 80:793-806, 1989.

77. Kapoor WN, Karpf M, Wieand S, Petereson JR, Levey GS. A prospective evaluation of follow-up of patients with syncope. N Engl J Med 309:197-204, 1983.

78. Gang ES, Peter T, Rosenthal ME, Mandel WJ, Lass Y. Detection of late potentials on the surface electrocardiogram in unexplained syncope. Am J Cardiol 58:1014-1020, 1986.

79. Winters SL, Stewart D, Gomes JA. Signal averaging of the surface QRS complex predicts inducibility of ventricular tachycardia in patients with syncope of unknown origin: A prospective study. J Am Coll Cardiol 10:775-781, 1987.

80. LaCroix D, Dubuc M, Kus T, Savard P, Shenasa M, Nadeau R. Evaluation of arrhythmic causes of syncope: Correlation between Holter monitoring, electrophysiologic testing, and body surface potential mapping. Am Heart J 122:1346-1354, 1991.

81. Mehta D, Camm AJ. Signal-averaged electrocardiogram and significance of late potentials in patients with idiopathic ventricular tachycardia: A review. Clin Cardiol 12:307-312, 1989.

82. Kinoshita O, Fontaine G, Rosas F, Elias J, Iwa T, Tonet J, Lascault G, Frank R. Time and frequency domain analyses of the signal-averaged ECG in patients with arrhythmogenic right ventricular dysplasia. Circulation 91:715-721, 1995.

83. Cripps TR, Counihan PJ, Frenneaux MP, Ward DE, Camm AJ, McKenna WJ. Signal-averaged electrocardiography in hypertrophic cardiomyopathy. J Am Coll Cardiol 15:956-961, 1990.

84. Zimmerman M, Friedli B, Adamec R, Oberhänsli. Ventricular late potentials and induced ventricular arrhythmias after surgical repair of tetralogy of Fallot. Am J Cardiol 67:873-878, 1991.

85. Jabi H, Burger AJ, Orawiec B, Touchon RC. Late potentials in mitral valve prolapse. Am Heart J 122:1340-1345, 1991.

86. Milner MR, Hawley RJ, Jachim M, Lindsay J, Fletcher RD. Ventricular late potentials in myotonic dystrophy. Ann Intern Med 115:607-613, 1991.

7

Case Studies

The following case descriptions incorporate SAECG results into the management of a variety of clinical presentations. These examples are based on actual patient profiles and are intended to illustrate how one uses the SAECG along with other historical, noninvasive, and invasive findings.

Case Study #1 *(Figure 7.1)*

A 69-year-old female presents to the hospital 5 hours after onset of epigastric discomfort. Admission ECG is consistent with large anterior wall MI and t-PA is given. The hospital course is complicated by mild congestive heart failure, easily controlled by diuretics. The LVEF by MUGA is 22% with a large apical aneurysm. Her medications include furosemide, enalapril, and coumadin. An SAECG is performed prior to discharge on day 14 post-MI.

The patient's clinical course suggests a large infarcted region with significant clinical and laboratory evidence of left ventricular dysfunction. This alone would suggest a substantial risk of lethal ventricular arrhythmias. The SAECG is abnormal; the fQRS is mildly prolonged, and there is a demonstrable late potential. The presence of the abnormal SAECG predicts an even greater risk of serious arrhythmic events in follow-up than predicted by the LVEF. The risk is increased approximately sixfold, clearly placing this patient in a high-risk category; she is also a candidate for appropriate preventive therapy. Note that all three individual leads show similar degrees of abnormality as the vector composite lead.

Case Study #2 *(Figure 7.1)*

Same patient as in case study #1, 6 weeks later. This is the third outpatient visit. Patient explains that she was watching TV

147

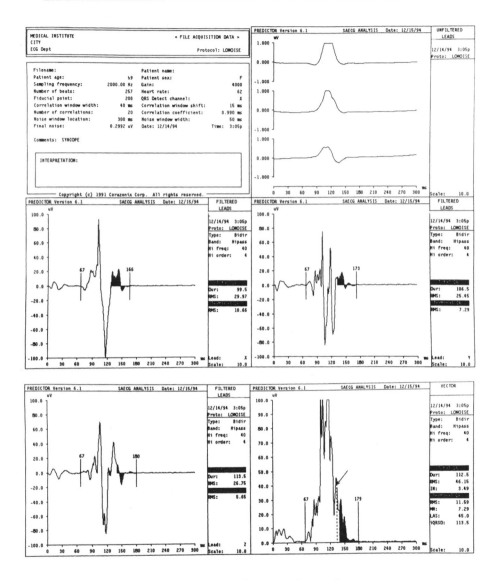

Figure 7.1. Case 1 and case 2.

when she suddenly felt weak and became diaphoretic. Symptoms lasted less than 1 minute. Holter monitor reveals normal sinus rhythm with rare ventricular premature depolarizations.

This patient had been previously identified as having a heightened risk for serious arrhythmic outcome. Beta-blocker therapy, known to reduce this risk especially in high-risk individuals, was presumably not used because of congestive heart failure. The noninvasive risk index was high and the patient's physicians were sensitive to the development of warning arrhythmias and so alerted the patient and his family. When she experienced a near syncopal event, she was brought to medical attention promptly. She was hospitalized on a monitored unit. The absence of ventricular ectopy on Holter offered no consolation as it is frequently unrewarding in the work-up of patients such as the one described here. Ventricular tachycardia was considered the most likely diagnosis and an early EPS in fact revealed sustained monomorphic VT that duplicated the clinical event.

Case Study #3 *(Figure 7.2)*

An 80-year-old female presents at hospital 2 hours after onset of severe substernal chest pain. ECG reveals ST elevation in II, III, F, rV_3 and rV_4, and tall R wave in V_1 and V_2. She is rushed to the cath lab where an occluded right coronary artery is opened by PTCA. Her recovery is uneventful. On day 10, a 2D echo shows mild hypokinesis of base of the inferior wall with overall EF >50% and normal right ventricular function. His medications on discharge were aspirin and metoprolol.

This patient apparently was in the process of progressing to a large inferior-posterior MI with right ventricular involvement when prompt primary angioplasty restored perfusion. The MI was largely aborted as evidenced by the near-normal LVEF. The SAECG was performed as part of the risk stratification process prior to hospital discharge. Although risk is clearly lower because of the well-preserved left ventricular function, the presence of some scar can create the substrate for life-threatening ventricular arrhythmias that can be predicted by the SAECG. In this case, a high-quality SAECG reveals a normal result in all leads including the vector. The fQRS is quite short, indicating a very low likelihood for arrhythmic events. This is particularly true, given that the site of MI was inferior, which would tend to accentuate any SAECG abnormality if present. The patient was appropriately treated and required no additional intervention.

Case Study #4 *(Figure 7.3)*

An elderly male experiences an acute MI while traveling. He has an uneventful hospitalization and returns home to his primary physician. The ECG reveals Q waves in V_2–V_5. The echo reveals

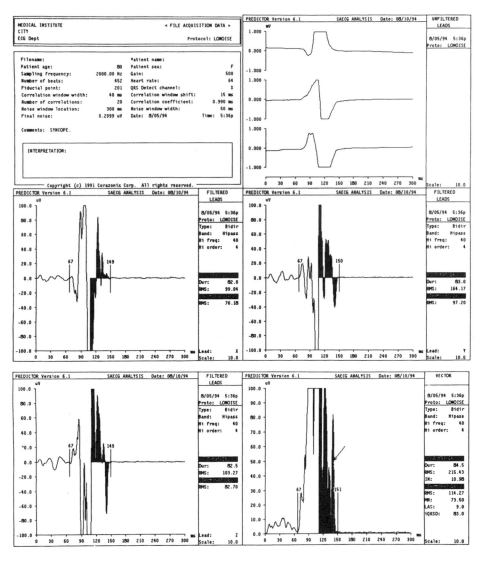

Figure 7.2. Case 3.

severe hypokinesis of the anterior wall and septum; overall EF is estimated at 40%. A Holter is performed and reveals 100 ventricular premature depolarizations/hour and 30 episodes of nonsustained VT. Three runs of nonsustained VT are >10 beats; the longest run is 30 beats at 175 bpm. The patient reports no symptoms.

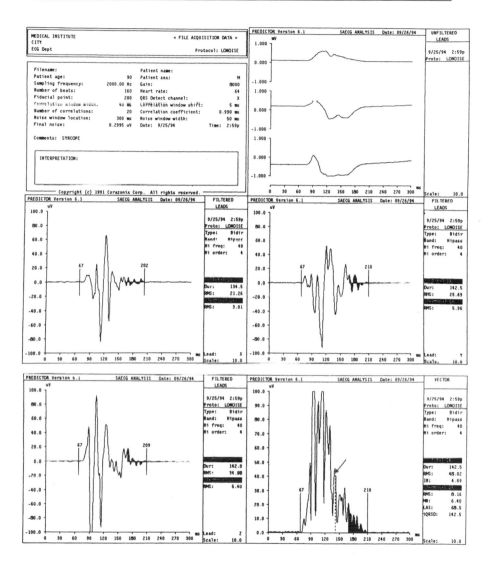

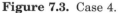

Figure 7.3. Case 4.

Figure 7.3 is a vector magnitude tracing of the SAECG. The tracing is high quality and reveals a markedly prolonged fQRS duration and clear evidence of a late potential, i.e., low V40 and prolonged low-amplitude signal. The magnitude of SAECG abnormality is particularly notable in the setting of previous anterior MI, which will tend to minimize the SAECG abnormality. The SAECG results imply greater risk of arrhythmic events during follow-up; the estimated risk based on fQRS alone would be in the range of 15% over the ensuing 12 months. The risk indicated by SAECG alone is further amplified by the presence of moderately severe left ventricular dysfunction and evidence of frequent and complex ventricular arrhythmia on the Holter ECG, as these results are independent of one another. Beta-blockers are clearly indicated, as the only indisputable treatment to prevent sudden death. Some physicians perform EPS in high-risk patients, especially given the presence of prolonged nonsustained VT.

Case Study #5 *(Figure 7.4)*

A 73-year-old female has been followed by your partner for 11 years since her anterior wall MI. She has done very well without angina or congestive heart failure. An exercise treadmill test last year was limited because of an orthopedic problem. The patient was playing with her grandchildren when she developed chest pressure, shortness of breath, and diaphoresis. She was rushed to the ER where ECG reveals a wide complex tachycardia; the systolic blood pressure is 100. Before any treatment could be given, normal sinus rhythm resumed spontaneously. Catheterization revealed three-vessel disease and LVEF of 42%. Your partner insists that the patient had ischemia-induced arrhythmia and plans CABG.

Figure 7.4 is an SAECG recorded well after MI. Note that it is recorded to a low noise level, and very low-amplitude QRS potentials can be visually sought because of the high quality of this recording. One notes that prior to filtering, even on averaged and amplified leads, no terminal QRS abnormalities can be observed. It is only after filtering and additional amplification that the individual leads can be clearly seen to have prominent late potentials and prolonged fQRS durations. Each lead is abnormal, which is the most typical pattern seen. The vector composite lead meets all criteria for SAECG abnormality; most importantly the fQRS is in a very prolonged range. The unfiltered QRS is not prolonged and the vector QRS prolongation is entirely attributed to the late potential that is invisible on the standard ECG. The clinical presentation also suggests that sustained VT is the mechanism responsible for the wide complex tachycardia. Although ischemia may play a role in the development of VT in this patient, the SAECG clearly indicates a markedly abnormal fixed substrate, a finding that also indicates permanent VT risk. EPS is usually performed to confirm the diagnostic suspicions and to help

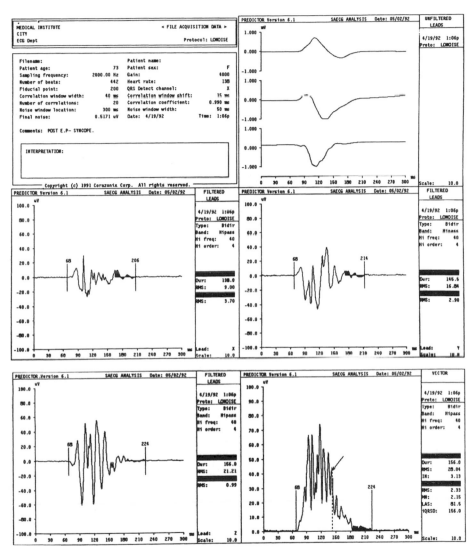

Figure 7.4. Case 5.

plan treatment options specific for VT, in addition to appropriate anti-ischemia therapy.

Case Study #6 *(Figure 7.5)*

A 69-year-old male with a remote MI and EF of 35% finds himself on the floor while preparing dinner. He is oriented but weak. One

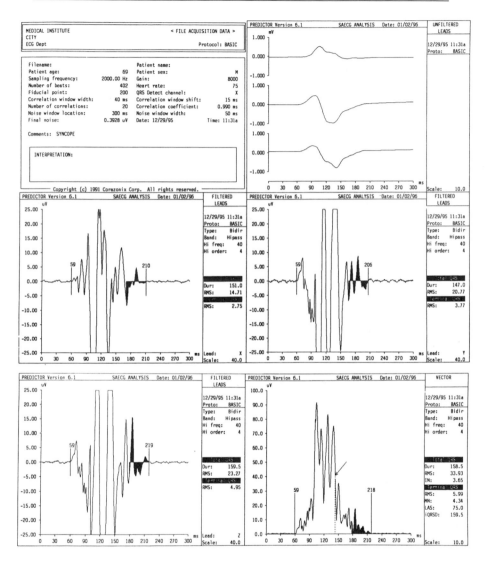

Figure 7.5. Case 6.

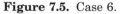

month later, while in your office, he casually mentions the event. He insists, however, that the episode was due to the glass of wine he had had, and his ACE inhibitor therapy.

This patient has had a prior MI and has experienced an episode of syncope. Although there are many causes of syncope, cardiac arrhythmias are common and an important diagnosis to consider. The most serious arrhythmic etiology, with dire prognostic implications if not recognized, diagnosed, and treated, is VT. The probability of VT as the cause of syncope in this patient is higher than average given the presence of a previous MI, but is not a certainty or even a likelihood. However, the SAECG result can shift the diagnostic probabilities substantially. This SAECG is clearly abnormal as indicated by the markedly prolonged fQRS. The combination of prior MI and an abnormal SAECG makes the diagnosis of VT a high probability; therefore, this patient requires prompt hospitalization and EPS.

Case Study #7 *(Figure 7.6)*

A 60-year-old businessman arrives from out of town and spends a hectic day, barely slowing down for coffee. That night, at dinner, he has two cocktails. Soon after starting dinner, he feels lighheaded and briefly loses consciousness. He awakens, feels nauseated and vomits, again briefly loses consciousness, and then is hospitalized under your care. He had CABG 7 years ago. He believes he had an MI, but is uncertain when questioned. The ECG reveals nonspecific ST/T wave abnormalities. An echocardiogram shows normal left ventricular wall motion.

This patient has coronary artery disease but not prior MI, an important distinction in terms of risk for VT. The SAECG is normal; the fQRS is not prolonged on the vector composite or the individual leads, and there is no late potential visible on a good quality tracing. The SAECG has excellent negative predictive accuracy for VT as presumed cause of syncope and thus this patient's risk of VT is low. Alternative diagnoses should be sought, and as suggested by the history, one possibility is neurally mediated syncope.

Case Study #8 *(Figure 7.7)*

A 43-year-old male is transferred after presenting with a wide complex tachycardia at a community hospital. The tachycardia had a left BBB and leftward axis morphology and a rate of 180 bpm. The patient tells you that the same thing happened 5 years ago when he was hospitalized at another hospital. You track down his workup, which revealed a "normal" echo and "normal" cath. He was discharged on quinidine and given the diagnosis of right ventricular outlet tract VT. The patient stopped his medication 2–3 years ago. The ECG reveals slightly tall R wave in V_1 and a QRS axis of +105°.

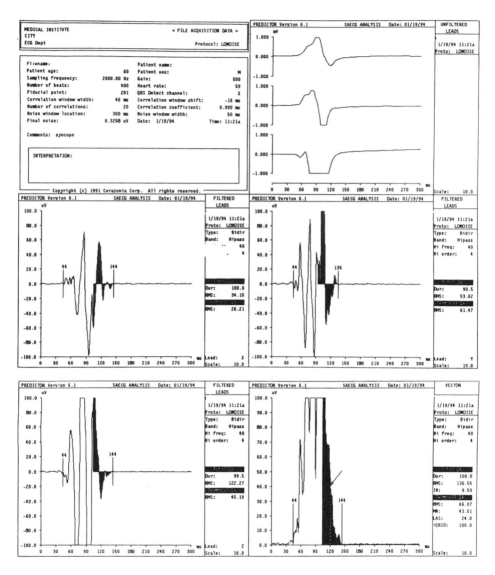

Figure 7.6. Case 7.

An echocardiogram is done and reveals normal left ventricular size and function and possible right ventricular dilation.

The SAECG recorded from this patient is strikingly abnormal and surely must influence one's thinking about this case. The fQRS duration of 163 msec is as long as one sees and more than a third

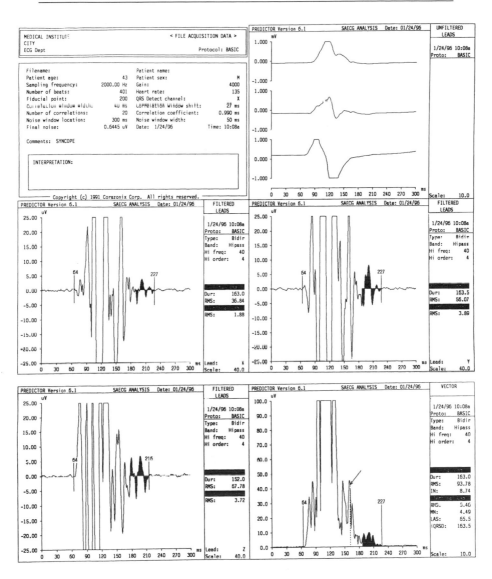

Figure 7.7. Case 8.

of the QRS is late potential. The SAECG is not abnormal for all
forms of supraventricular tachycardia when the QRS on standard
ECG is not abnormal (e.g., preexcited or BBB), thereby making supraventricular tachycardia with aberrancy an improbable diagnosis.
Left BBB tachycardias suggest an origin in the right ventricle in this

case when there is no evidence of left ventricular cardiomyopathy or MI. These are unusual VTs and raise several considerations. Idiopathic VTs usually originiate in the right ventricular outlet tract but virtually always have normal SAECG results. However, VT in the setting of arrhythmogenic right ventricular dysplasia (or other right ventricular cardiomyopathies) will also cause left BBB tachycardias. These patients almost always have conduction delay visible on the SAECG. The SAECG in this case pointed the physicians in the right direction to detect underlying structural heart disease; a right ventricular angiogram and an MRI were diagnostic of ARVD, a diagnosis with more serious prognostic implications than idiopathic VT from the right ventricular outlet tract.

Case Study #9 *(Figure 7.8)*

A 56-year-old postwoman is delivering mail to the local internist when he collapses. A "quick-look" ECG reveals ventricular fibrillation and the patient is defibrillated. ECG immediately after reveals 3–4 mm ST elevation in V_1–V_4. At the hospital, repeat ECG reveals that the ST elevation had returned to baseline. CK increases to 300 (normal <120). Cath reveals severe proximal LAD stenosis. There is questionable anterior wall hypokinesis.

The SAECG recorded soon after this patient's near fatal event is normal. A normal result suggests a lower likelihood of VT, which may be due to the absence of substrate for VT. In this case, there is evidence of an acute and severe ischemic event culminating in cardiac arrest but no evidence of previous MI scar. An acute and reversible cause of VF will not be reflected on the SAECG unless permanent damage results. Treatment in these cases is usually aimed at the inciting ischemic lesion with revascularization.

Case Study #10 *(Figure 7.9)*

A 73-year-old female with a history of two previous MIs is followed by you. She has had intermittent congestive heart failure; the EF is 30%. She presents to another hospital with a wide complex tachycardia at 150 bpm. She is given procainamide and 1 hour later normal sinus rhythm resumes. ECG reveals normal sinus rhythm, poor R wave progression, and Q waves in leads III, and aVF. Only a single lead of the wide complex tachycardia is available and analysis is nondiagnostic. EPS reveals no inducible VT. You are greatly concerned regarding the uncertainty of the diagnosis.

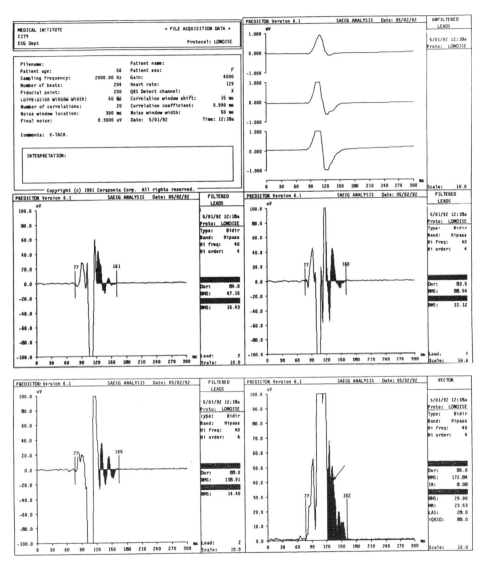

Figure 7.8. Case 9.

Clearly, this patient has an elevated risk of VT. When evaluating a patient with these clinical characteristics and a wide complex tachycardia, VT was and should be the primary diagnosis until proven otherwise. The EPS is the gold standard for the diagnosis of VT and has a very high sensitivity when the arrhythmia has occurred

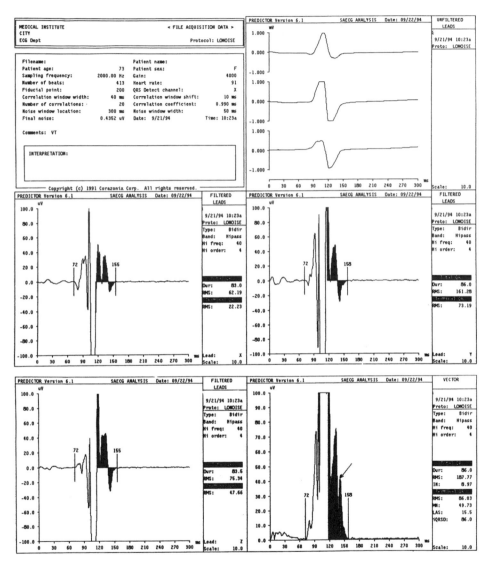

Figure 7.9. Case 10.

clinically. The negative EPS disturbed the physicians because of the concern of a missed VT diagnosis. The SAECG in this case reveals no abnormality; the fQRS duration and terminal voltage and duration are well within the normal range. Because the SAECG is also highly sensitive for the diagnosis of VT in the setting of coronary heart disease, it is confirmatory to the EPS results. A repeat EPS subsequently revealed atrial flutter with 2:1 atrioventricular conduction and QRS aberration.

Case Study #11 *(Figure 7.10)*

A 87-year-old female is referred to your office for syncope and an abnormal SAECG. The ECG reveals normal sinus rhythm, first degree atrioventricular block, and left BBB.

The SAECG in this case is markedly abnormal by fQRS duration criteria. However, the presence of left BBB precludes accurate interpretation of the SAECG and its clinical implications. It is important to recognize the presence of BBB or severe intraventricular conduction defect before SAECG analysis.

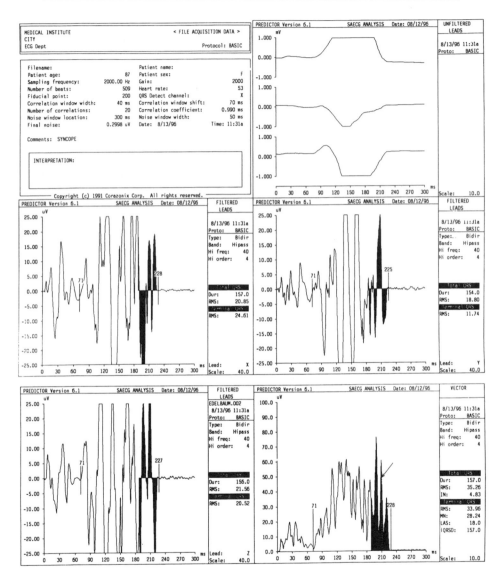

Figure 7.10. Case 11.

8

Future Applications of the High-Resolution Electrocardiogram

New Methods and Applications

The incorporation of new technology for recording cardiac activity is a natural progression that has occurred since the earliest days of electrocardiography. From the string galvanometer to the vacuum tube to the transistor to the integrated circuit to the embedded computer, this evolution was for the most part focused on signals that were observed almost a century ago. The advent of computing technology elevated the process to one of automating a manual process, such as waveform amplitude and time interval measurements. Today, the software manipulation of the ECG allows the observation of signals heretofore deemed inaccessible, e.g., His-Purkinje potentials, as well as signals previously unknown, e.g., late potentials. As more is learned about the nature of myocardial activation, particularly in diseased states, the application of newer techniques will further aid in noninvasive diagnosis. Following are three such new applications.

High-resolution analysis of the P wave brings new noninvasive tools to the analysis of atrial activation. Once viewed in high-resolution mode, the P wave can no longer be considered just a small rounded "bump" that precedes the QRS. The P wave is a rich-appearing waveform and initial observations are very promising for identifying patients prone to atrial fibrillation.

A significant aspect of traditional late potential analysis that has been recognized but not well studied is the fact that not all abnormally activated regions around an infarct will outlast the QRS complex and hence result in late potentials. There are known differences in late potential manifestations between anterior and inferior infarcts due to the normally activated ventricular sequence where the left anterior wall will activate sooner than the inferior regions of the left ventricle. Hence, late activation of viable cells within and surrounding an anterior infarct will be less likely to outlast the QRS than similar regions in the inferior wall. This difference aside, there is still the likelihood that not all abnormal regions will have depolarizing cells that will always outlast the QRS complex. Identifying these abnormal potentials that overlap in time with the QRS complex is indeed a challenging problem.

The high-resolution ECG has been primarily implemented with signal averaging where each beat is considered of equal weight and the average is the result of this uniformly weighted measurement of an unbiased estimate of the mean. However, if one can identify special characteristics of the signals of interest and the interfering noise, there may be ways to use this information before applying the averaging process. Such an optimal filter will produce a biased estimate of the mean. Initial studies have shown that this approach will result in a low-noise recording requiring far fewer beats than a typical signal-averaged recording. Such a reduction of the number of beats needed to obtain a valid recording may open new study opportunities such as recordings during balloon inflation of an angioplasty procedure, or immediately post exercise while the subject's heart rate is still elevated.

Following are brief overviews of these three applications of the high-resolution ECG.

P Wave Analysis

The most common arrhythmia in clinical practice and the most frequent arrhythmic diagnosis leading to hospitalization is atrial fibrillation (AF). AF can be benign, isolated, and short-lived in some instances, and in others, it can be the root cause of serious cardiovascular complications including stroke and death. The prevalence of AF increases with age; it is rare in young patients but occurs in as many as 5% of patients older than 60 years of age. AF may develop when there are no detectable structural abnormalities and is then characterized as lone or idiopathic AF. More frequently, AF is a complication of underlying heart disease such as hypertension and coronary artery disease.

AF is a reentrant arrhythmia; it is not the result of a single circuit as most other arrhythmias but instead depends on the presence of several simultaneous and nonstationary circuits present in atrial tissue. The number, size, route, and stability of the reentrant circuits are determined by the electrophysiological characteristics of the atrial myocardium. AF can only persist if a minimum number of circuits (also called wavelets) are maintained. Both conduction velocity and tissue refractoriness will operate in concert to determine the susceptibility of an individual to AF.[1] Altering conditions prevalent in atrial myocardium can be viewed as either proarrhythmic or antiarrhythmic depending on the effects of conduction velocity or refractoriness. Most germane to signal averaging, when conduction is slowed, AF is more likely to develop or persist. Both intra-atrial conduction delay and atrial electrographic fragmentation have been associated with greater risk of AF and support the concept described above. The importance of conduction delay to AF underlies the central conceptual and technical processes that led to the development of SAECG recording of the P wave.

For signal averaging of the P wave, the acquisition is performed with the patients in sinus rhythm. In order to average the P wave, one must recognize that the relationship between P wave and QRS is nonfixed and will vary slightly from beat to beat because of the respiratory cycle and variations in autonomic tone. The changes in vagal tone responsible for sinus arrhythmia will also alter the PR interval. If the signal-averaging process is using an R wave triggered system without making specific concessions to the varying PR interval, the averaged P wave will be affected, resulting in loss of high-frequency energy, a result known as jitter. To overcome this potential limitation, the acquisition process can utilize one of two approaches: a second trigger can be used to align the P wave after averaging has been initiated by an R wave trigger[2] or a strict beat rejection system can guard against acceptance of any beats that are not properly aligned with a preselected sinus P wave.[3] Both have been used successfully in clinical studies; the second approach can be programmed on systems that are not specifically designed for signal averaging of the P wave.

With the averaging system appropriately adjusted for P wave acquisition, the averaging of the P wave proceeds in a similar fashion to QRS averaging. The lead systems are similar and the endpoint of averaging is low noise, e.g., 0.3 μV. The noise window should be appropriately shifted to reflect the pre-P wave interval for sampling. The acquisition tends to be slower than QRS acquisition because more beats are rejected to achieve high-quality fits with the template P wave rather than for the sole purpose of noise reduction. A typical average might run approximately 20 minutes.

Once the P wave has been averaged, the complex is filtered and processed; most commonly, a vector magnitude is used to reflect the global atrial activation pattern and is shown in Figure 8.1. Various filters have been used successfully, although some filters and filter bandwidths may be more advantageous than others.[4] Clinical studies with the P wave SAECG have used both total duration of the P wave as well as "atrial late potentials" or terminal P wave amplitude measurements. The total duration is consistently useful, but there is uncertainty regarding the clinical and pathophysiological validity of terminal measurements.[4]

Several initial studies were recently reported and indicated the potential value of the P wave SAECG.[2,3,5] All enrolled primarily patients with paroxysmal AF; methodology differed somewhat from study to study. It was important to exclude patients who are using antiarrhythmic agents (primarily class 1 and amiodarone) because these may lengthen atrial activation unpredictably.

In a case control study where patients were matched prior to entry, the P wave SAECG was contrasted with the standard ECG in its association with prior AF.[3] In 15 patients with AF, the unfiltered and filtered P wave durations from individual orthogonal leads and the filtered vector magnitude were all significantly longer than in the matched controls without AF. The standard ECG limb lead II P wave duration did not demonstrate this difference. The differentiation between AF and control patients was enhanced by filtering; this may be due to better visualization of the onset and offset of the P wave, enhanced detection of terminal low-amplitude P wave components, or the filter itself. Figure 8.2 illustrates the difference between patients (hashed bars) and controls (solid bars) in the XYZ leads and the filtered vector magnitude. The vector P wave duration was approximately 16 msec longer (20%) in the AF patients than in the controls: 162 ± 15 msec versus 140 ± 12 msec (p<0.01). Values of P wave duration were selected and had good discriminating value; for example, a P wave duration of >155 msec predicted AF with a sensitivity of 80% and a specificity of 93%.

An important study by Fukunami et al.[2] demonstrated that a P wave-triggered SAECG was technically feasible and yielded relevant data on the signal-averaged P wave. A total of 42 patients with paroxysmal AF and 50 matched controls were analyzed; patients with AF were characterized by longer P wave duration on the SAECG and lower terminal voltage of the P wave ("atrial late potential"). Interestingly, neither the P wave duration on the standard ECG nor

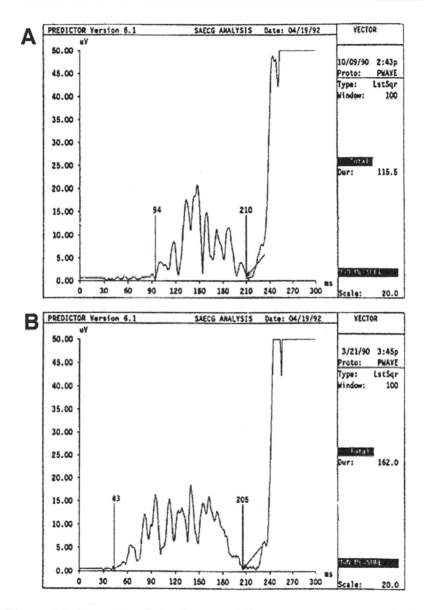

Figure 8.1. Examples of signal-averaged P-waves on a vector magnitude tracing. Panel **A** is from a control patient (duration = 116 msec) and panel **B** is from a patient with recent AF (duration = 162 msec). Lst Sqr = least fit filter; proto = protocol. (Reprinted with permission from JACC; Guidera SA and Steinberg JS.[3])

P wave duration (ms)

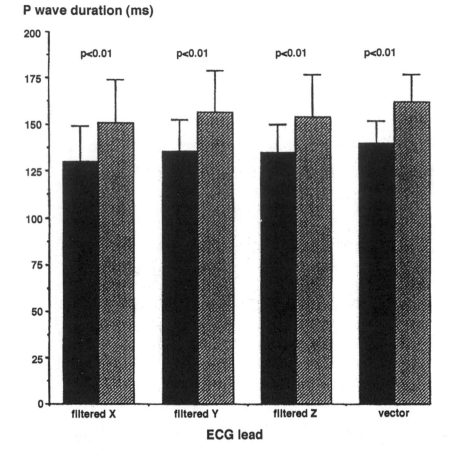

Figure 8.2. The filtered P-wave duration in patients with AF (hashed bars) and controls (solid bars) in the XYZ leads and the filtered vector magnitude. A duration of ≥155 msec identified patients with a history of AF with a sensitivity of 80% and a specificity of 93%. (Reprinted with permission from JACC; Guidera SA, and Steinberg JS.[3])

the left atrial dimension on two-dimensional echocardiogram was capable of distinguishing AF patients from the controls.

Iwakura et al.[6] reported that the filtered P wave duration in patients with more frequent attacks (once a month or more) of paroxysmal AF was significantly longer than in those with less frequent episodes (140 ± 14 msec versus 131 ± 11 msec). Recently the same group demonstrated prospectively the utility of P wave SAECG in predicting the transition of paroxysmal AF to chronic AF. They defined P wave SAECG with a filtered P wave duration of ≥145 msec and root mean square voltage for the last 30 msec (LP30) < 3.0 μV as abnormal. In 123 patients with paroxysmal AF followed for a mean period of 26 ± 12 months, 43% of patients with abnormal P wave SAECG as compared to only 4% of patients with normal SAECG developed chronic AF.

The results of the P wave SAECG appear to have a strong relationship to the development of postoperative AF following cardiac surgery.[7-9] Interestingly, the risk in this setting is based on a preoperative finding, the P wave duration on the SAECG. Risk was increased approximately fourfold when the P wave was prolonged and was independent of other clinical variables.[7] Because AF remains a frequent problem after cardiac surgery, contributing to hospital length of stay[10] and morbidity, identification of high-risk patients with a targeted therapeutic approach may be a logical outcome of these data.

The P wave analysis from the SAECG has recently been used to predict recurrent AF after successful catheter ablation of the Wolff-Parkinson-White syndrome[11] and to better understand the effect of increased atrial size on atrial conduction.[12] The P wave SAECG will likely see increasing use as a noninvasive representation of atrial conduction and as a probe into the mechanisms of AF in a variety of clinical settings.

Abnormal Intra-QRS Potentials

In the normal heart one can assume that activation of the ventricular myocardium is a deterministic event, that is, one that proceeds in a predictable fashion on a beat-to-beat basis. Also, once activated, then propagation in the ventricles occurs from region to region in a "smooth," continuous fashion. In other words, activation wavefronts do not abruptly stop or change directions as might be the case when an infarcted region is present. In the latter case, the transition from viable to dead tissue may not be strictly demarcated as in the case of a mottled infarct. Experimental arrhythmia models using induced infarcts in canines are the primary method for studying many ventricular arrhythmias. Cardiac mapping studies, which utilize hundreds of recording sites from all regions of the ventricles, describe the sequence of activation in the regions of the electrode placements. Figure 8.3 is an example of 30 such recordings from the epicardial region overlying an infarct region in a canine infarction model. The left group of electrograms appears to be from a normal region and has the characteristic biphasic appearance of a unipolar

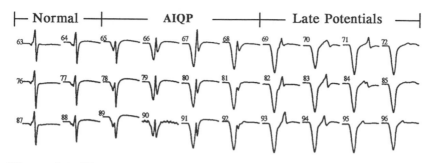

Figure 8.3. These 30 electrograms obtained from the epicardium over a canine infarct demonstrate three distinct electrogram types. On the left are normal, biphasic recordings. In the center, the electrograms have discrete abnormal intra-QRS potentials (AIQP), and on the right the Q waves over the infarct are followed by a late potential deflection.

recording. By visually tracking the electrograms from left to right, one can observe a distinct change in the normal biphasic electrogram with the appearance of another mid-QRS deflection. This region is labeled AIQP for abnormal intra-QRS potential. On the right side the electrograms show a deep Q wave indicative of an infarct, but following the QRS is a discrete deflection in most of these electrograms. These are the direct recordings of the cardiac late potentials that would be recorded with the standard SAECG. However, the AIQP signals would not be readily discernable since they would be masked within the QRS when recorded at the body surface.

A sophisticated approach to separating the AIQP from the QRS complex involves a mathematical modeling approach.[13] This approach uses an autoregressive model of the QRS that creates a "smoothed" version of the QRS from which the original QRS is subtracted. This difference results in a residual signal that can be quantified and used to stratify patients much like a late potential study.[14] Figure 8.4 demonstrates the result of this approach in two patients. Panel A is from a patient with ventricular tachycardia and a normal duration QRS of 92 msec. The solid line is the original signal-averaged QRS complex. The dotted line is the modeled QRS. Beneath these two signals is the difference or residual signal with the AIQP labeled. Panel B is from a patient who did not have a ventricular tachycardia and also with a QRSd of 92 msec. There is no similar amplitude AIQP signal in this patient. In a data set of 173 patients previously analyzed with traditional methods, the quantification of the AIQP improved the specificity from 89% to 95% and the positive predictive value increased from 25% to 47%.[14]

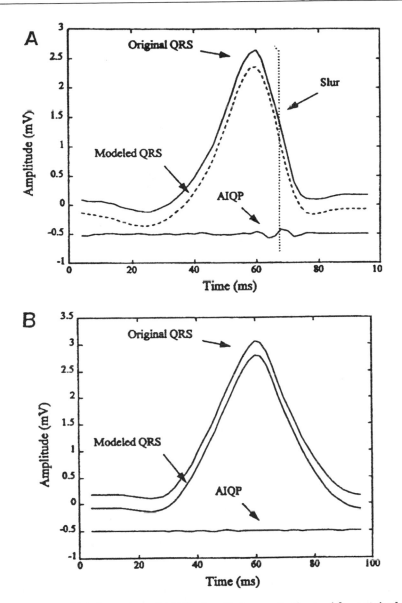

Figure 8.4. The detection of AIQP signals from a patient with ventricular tachycardia is shown in panel **A**. The original QRS signal is a solid line and the modeled QRS is a dotted line. The difference is where the AIQP are observable in the bottom trace. Panel **B**, in the same format as panel **A**, is from a patient without ventricular tachycardia and the relative absence of an AIQP signal. (Reprinted with permission of the American Heart Association; Lander P, et al.[14])

Optimal Filtering

Spectral estimation methods were discussed in Chapter 4, and while the rationale was very strong for this approach, it was pointed out that the there are serious limitations for estimating the frequency spectra using current approaches. However, this does not rule out the use of frequency domain approaches when the goal is not quantifying the spectral content of the signal but using the frequency domain representation to perform certain mathematical functions. Once these mathematical operations are performed, the signal can be transformed back to the time domain to observe the results of these manipulations. One such method is to create an optimal filter based on the spectral content of the noise and the signal. This filter may change on a beat-to-beat basis and its primary function is to suppress the noise component of the signal while minimally altering the desired signal. After each filtering operation, the signal is then averaged in the conventional manner. In practice, this type of filter will produce a biased estimate of the signal average and the signal may not appear identical to the unbiased estimate of the nonfiltered approach. Its advantage is that the signal-to-noise ratio can be increased with far fewer beats than without the optimal filter. The theoretical basis of this approach goes into great detail about the methods that are beyond the scope of this presentation.[15,16] In a clinical application,[17] the optimal filtering method using 64 beats was compared with the standard approach of increasing the number of beats in an average until the noise falls below 0.03 μV.

Figure 8.5 shows examples of signal-averaged data from the same patient. Panel A is a 64-beat average without any special filtering. One possible role for traditional low-pass filtering is to attempt to separate signal and noise. The use of 100-Hz low-pass filtering and averaging for 64 beats is shown in panel B. In both panels A and B, the QRS$_{offset}$ does not appear to detect any late potential components. In panel A, the QRSd is 104 msec and in panel B the QRSd 102 msec. The shaded region, which depicts the late potentials, is within the body of the QRS complex. Panel C was obtained by averaging 64 beats that were optimally filtered. Note the appearance of the late potentials by the shaded region and a QRSd of 147 msec. Panel D was obtained by averaging 900 beats, without any special filters, resulting in a noise reduction to 0.3 μV. Note the late potentials in the shaded region and a QRSd of 143 msec. Thus the 64-beat optimally filtered signal average (panel D) is almost identical to the low-noise traditional average (panel D).

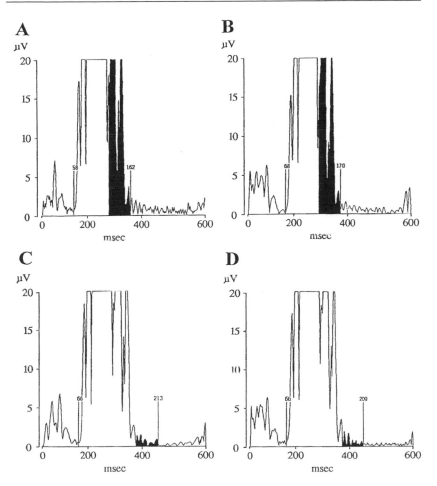

Figure 8.5. The detection of late potentials is not obvious in panels **A** and **B** where 64 beats are averaged. In panel **B** there was an additional 100-Hz low-pass filter. Panel **C** is the average of the same 64 beats as in panels **A** and **B**, but after the inclusion of an optimal filter to selectively reduce noise. Panel **D** was obtained by averaging 900 beats in the typical fashion and noise was reduced to 0.3 μV. (Reprinted with permission of the American Heart Association; Lander P, et al.[17])

Note, however, that the late potentials do not have the same morphology in these two panels. This is the difference of the biased estimator (panel C) with the unbiased estimator (panel D). The utility of this optimal approach has yet to be determined in multiple or large-scale studies.

References

1. Allessie MA, Lammers WJ, Hollen J, et al. Experimental evaluation of Moe's multiple wavelet hypothesis of atrial fibrillation. In: Zipes D, Jalife J (eds). Cardiac Electrophysiology Arrhythmias, Grune & Stratton, New York, pp 265-275, 1985.
2. Fukunami M, Yamada T, Hoki N, et al. Detection of patients at risk for paroxysmal atrial fibrillation during sinus rhythm by P wave triggered signal averaged electrocardiogram. Circulation 83:162-169, 1991.
3. Guidera SA, Steinberg JS. The signal averaged P wave duration: A rapid and noninvasive marker of risk of atrial fibrillation. J Am Coll Cardiol 21:1645-1651, 1993.
4. Ehlert FA, Korenstein D, Steinberg JS. Evaluation of P-wave signal-averaged electrocardiographic filtering and analysis methods. Am Heart J 134:985-993, 1997.
5. Stafford PJ, Turner I, Vincent R. Quantitative analysis of signal averaged P waves in idiopathic paroxysmal atrial fibrillation. J Am Coll Cardiol 21:181A, 1993.
6. Iwakura K, Abe Y, Fukunami M, et al. Relationship between frequency and duration of paroxysmal atrial fibrillation attacks and atrial late potentials. Circulation 86(Suppl I):I-130, 1992.
7. Steinberg JS, Zelenkofske S, Wong SC, Gelernt M, Sciacca R, Menchavez E. Value of the P-wave signal-averaged ECG for predicting atrial fibrillation after cardiac surgery. Circulation 88:2618-2622, 1993.
8. Hutchinson LA, Steinberg JS. Prospective study of atrial fibrillation after cardiac surgery: Multivariate risk analysis using P wave signal-averaged ECG and clinical variables. Ann Noninv Elec 1:133-140, 1996.
9. Klein M, Blumberg S, Bodenheimer MM, et al. Use of P wave triggered signal averaged ECG to predict atrial fibrillation after coronary artery bypass surgery. Am Heart J 129:895-901, 1995.
10. Tamis JE, Steinberg JS. Atrial fibrillation is the only modifiable factor that lengthens hospital stay after coronary artery bypass surgery. PACE 19:622A, 1996.
11. Maia IG, Filho FESC, Fagundes MLA, Boghossian SH, Vanheusden L, Sa RM, Alves PAG. Signal-averaged P wave in patients with Wolff-Parkinson-White syndrome after successful radiofrequency catheter ablation. J Am Coll Cardiol 26:1310-1314, 1995.
12. Keller AM, Steinberg JS, Abreu JE, Gopal AS, King DL. Signal-averaged P wave duration: Relation to atrial volume as assessed by cine magnetic resonance imaging. Circulation 92:I-407, 1995.
13. Gomis P, Jones DL, Caminal P, Berbari EJ, Lander P. Analysis of abnormal signal within the QRS complex of the high-resolution electrocardiogram. IEEE Trans Biomed Eng 44:681-693, 1997.
14. Lander P, Gomis P, Goyal R, Berbari EJ, Caminal P, Lazzara R, Steinberg JS. Analysis of intra-QRS late potentials: Improved predictive value for arrhythmic events using the signal-averaged electrocardiogram. Circulation 95:1386-1393, 1997.
15. Lander P, Berbari EJ. Time-frequency plane Weiner filtering of the high resolution ECG: Background and time-frequency representations. IEEE Trans Biomed Eng 44:247-255, 1997.

16. Lander P, Berbari EJ. Time-frequency plane Weiner filtering of the high resolution ECG: Development and application. IEEE Trans Biomed Eng 44:256-265, 1997.
17. Lander P, Berbari EJ, Lazzara R. Optimal filtering and quality control of the signal-averaged electrocardiogram: Hi-fidelity 1-minute recordings. Circulation 91:1495-1505, 1995.

Index

Ablation, surgical, 16-17
Abnormal intra-QRS potentials, 169-170, 171
Abnormal ventricular activation during normal sinus rhythm, 8-10
A/D converter, 28, 29
Advanced heart failure, 122-127
Age and signal-averaged electrocardiogram interpretation, 65
Algorithms, automatic measurement, 70-71, 72
Alignment of late potentials, 30-34
Ambulatory electrocardiogram, 65-70
Amplitude of late potential, 16
Analog filtering of signal-averaged electrocardiogram, 65-70
Analysis of signal-averaged electrocardiogram, 41-61
digital filtering in, 43-50
frequency domain, 58-60
individual lead, 55-58
vector magnitude in, 50-55
Antiarrhythmic drugs and late potentials, 76-77, 78
Arrhythmic events, spontaneous, 87-88

Arrhythmogenic right ventricular dysplasia, 137
Artifacts, 77-80
Automatic measurement algorithms, 70-71, 72

BBB; See Bundle branch block
Beat detection of late potentials, 30-34
Bidirectional filter, 48-50
Body surface, late potentials recorded on, 21-40; See also Late potentials
Bundle branch block, 76, 77
Butterworth filter, 48

Cardiac death, sudden, 3-4, 138
Cardiomyopathy, idiopathic dilated, 122-127
nonsustained ventricular tachycardia and, 127-129
Case studies, 147-161
Clinical practice, 83-145
arrhythmia prediction in, 94-103
arrhythmogenic right ventricular dysplasia in, 137
establishing utility of electrocardiogram in, 83

177

idiopathic dilated cardiomyopathy and nonsustained
ventricular tachycardia
in, 127-129
introduction to, 83-87
nonsustained ventricular
tachycardia in, 118-122
prognostic value in, 122-127
programmed ventricular
stimulation in, 107-118
risk prediction in, 88-94,
103-105
spontaneous arrhythmic
events in, 87-88
sudden cardiac death in,
138
surgically repaired tetralogy
of Fallot in, 138-139
technical and clinical limitations in, 105-106
unexplained syncope in,
129-136
ventricular tachycardia in,
136-137
Computers, 29-30
Conduction defects, intraventricular, 76, 77
Conduction delay, 7-19
abnormal ventricular activation in, 8-10
late potential and, 10-17
sustained ventricular tachycardia in, 7-8
Converter, 28, 29
Correlation of QRS complex,
31-33

Data acquisition for late potential recording, 28, 29
Death, sudden cardiac, 3-4,
138

Digital filtering of signal-averaged electrocardiogram, 43-
50
late potential identification,
65-70
Dilated cardiomyopathy, idiopathic, 122-127
nonsustained ventricular
tachycardia and, 127-129
Displaying of signal-averaged
electrocardiogram, 39
Duration of late potential, 16

Electrically induced ventricular tachycardia, 129-136
Endocardial recording and delayed conduction, 14-15
Epicardial recording and delayed conduction, 14-15
Experimental infarction and
delayed conduction, 10-17

Fast Fourier transform, 59
FFT; *See* Fast Fourier
transform
Fibrous scar tissue, 8-10
delayed conduction and, 14
Filtered vector magnitude
automatic measurement al-
gorithms and, 70-71, 72
in noise calculation, 35-37
parameters derived from,
50-55
XYZ leads and, 41-42
Filtering, 25-28
digital, 43-50
in late potential identification, 65-70
optimal, 172-173
Fourier analysis, 59
Fractionated electrogram

delayed electrical activity and, 12

in healed myocardial infarction, 10

Fragmented electrogram, 14-15

Frequency domain analysis, 58-60

Future applications, 163-175

abnormal intra-QRS potentials in, 169-170, 171

optimal filtering in, 172-173

P wave analysis in, 164-169

Gender and signal-averaged electrogram interpretation, 64-65

Graph in individual lead analysis, 55-58

Healing after myocardial infarction, 8-10

Heart disease, 136-139

Heart failure, advanced, 122-127

High-pass filtering of signal-averaged electrocardiogram, 65-70

High-resolution electrocardiogram, 1-5; *See also* Signal-averaged electrocardiogram

definition of, 1

future applications of, 163-175; *See also* Future applications

His-Purkinje system, 2

History of use of signal-averaged electrocardiogram, 83-87

Holter electrocardiogram, 65-70

Idiopathic dilated cardiomyopathy, 122-127

nonsustained ventricular tachycardia and, 127-129

prognostic value of signal-averaged electrocardiogram in patients, 122-127

Individual lead analysis, 55-58

Instrumentation for late potential recording, 24-28

Intra-QRS potentials, 169-170, 171

Intraventricular conduction defects, 76, 77

LAS duration; *See* Low-amplitude signal duration

Late potentials, 21-40

antiarrhythmic drugs and, 76-77, 78

conduction delay and, 10-17

data acquisition for, 28, 29

filtering in identification of, 65-70

instrumentation for, 24-28

lead systems for, 21-24

noise and measurement of, 71-76

recording of, 2-3, 4

signal averaging of, 29-39

Lead analysis of signal-averaged electrocardiogram, 55-58

Lead systems for late potential recording, 21-24

Low amplitude signal duration, 50-51, 55

Low-pass filtering, 65-70

MI; *See* Myocardial infarction

Myocardial conduction delay;
  See Conduction delay
Myocardial infarction
  abnormality early after, 87-88
  case studies of, 147-161
  case study of, 146
  first year after, 116-118
  predischarge risk stratification after, 88-94
  sustained ventricular tachycardia after, 7-8
  technical and clinical limitations after, 105-106
  ventricular activation and, 8-10
  ventricular arrhythmias after, 94-103

Necrosis, 8-10
  delayed conduction and, 14
Noise and late potentials, 14
  calculations of, 35-39
  measurement of, 71-76
Nomogram in individual lead analysis, 55-58
Nonsustained ventricular tachycardia
  idiopathic dilated cardiomyopathy and, 127-129
  sustained ventricular tachycardia and, 118-122
Normal signal-averaged electrocardiogram, problems, 63-81
  antiarrhythmic drugs and late potentials, 76
  artifacts and quality control, 77-80
  automatic measurement algorithms, 70-71

bundle branch block and intraventricular conduction defects, 76
effects of noise on late potential measurements, 71-76
filtering, role of, 65-70
Normal sinus rhythm, abnormal ventricular activation during, 8-10

Optimal filtering, 172-173

Post-averaging method
  in noise calculation, 35-37
  XYZ leads and, 41-42
Premature ventricular contraction, 31-33
Printing of signal-averaged electrocardiogram, 39
Programmed ventricular stimulation, 107-118
Propafenone and late potentials, 76-77, 78
PVC; *See* Premature ventricular contraction
P wave analysis, 164-169

QRS complex
  analysis of signal-averaged electrocardiogram and, 41-43
  automatic measurement algorithms and, 70-71, 72
  bidirectional filter and, 48-50
  bundle branch block and, 76, 77
  detection and alignment of, 30-34

filtered vector magnitude
and, 50-55
QRS duration
in analysis of signal-averaged electrocardiogram,
51
in frequency domain analysis, 58-60
in individual lead analysis,
55-58
signal-averaged electrocardiogram parameters and,
63-65
QRS potentials, abnormal,
169-170, 171
Quality control, 77-80

Recording late potentials on
the body surface, 21-40
Reentry
late potentials and, 17
in sustained ventricular
tachycardia, 7-8
Right ventricular dysplasia, arrhythmogenic, 137
Risk prediction
electrocardiogram as tool
for, 88-94
electrocardiogram variables
or components in, 103-105
RMS voltage; *See* Root mean
square voltage
Root mean square in noise calculation, 35-37
Root mean square voltage, 50-
55

SAECG; *See* Signal-averaged
electrocardiogram
Scar tissue, 8-10
delayed conduction and, 14

Signal-averaged electrocardiogram, 63-81
analysis of, 41-61; *See also*
Analysis of signal-aver-
aged electrocardiogram
antiarrhythmic drugs and,
76-77, 78
artifacts and, 77-80
automatic measurement al-
gorithms in, 70-71, 72
bundle branch block and,
76, 77
case studies of, 147-161; *See
also* Case studies
in clinical practice, 83-145;
See also Clinical practice
conduction delay detected
on, 7-19; *See also* Conduction delay
definition of, 1-2
filtering in, 65-70
noise and, 71-76
normal, 63-65
Signal averaging of late potentials, 29-39
Simson bidirectional filter, 48-
50
Sinusoidal composition of signals, 59
Sinus rhythm, abnormal ventricular activation during, 8-
10
Software, 29-30
Spontaneous arrhythmic
events, 87-88
Standard deviation in noise
calculation, 37-38
Storing of signal-averaged electrocardiogram, 39
Sudden cardiac death, 3-4,
138
Surgical ablation, 16-17

Surgically repaired tetralogy of Fallot, 138-139

Sustained ventricular tachycardia
    after myocardial infarction, 7-8
    inducibility of, 118-122

Syncope, 129-136

Tetralogy of Fallot, surgically repaired, 138-139

Thrombolytic therapy, 111-116

Unexplained syncope, 129-136

Vector magnitude
    in analysis of signal-averaged electrocardiogram, 50-55
    automatic measurement algorithms and, 70-71, 72
    in noise calculation, 35-37
    XYZ leads and, 41-42

Ventricular activation during normal sinus rhythm, 8-10

Ventricular arrhythmias after myocardial infarction, 87-88, 94-103

Ventricular dysplasia, arrhythmogenic right, 137

Ventricular fibrillation, 85-87

Ventricular tachycardia
    in clinical practice, 118-122
    nonsustained, 127-129
    predicting electrically induced, 129-136
    signal-averaged electrocardiogram in, 83-87
    sustained, 7-8
    syncope and, 129-136

VF; *See* Ventricular fibrillation

Voltage, root mean square, 50-55

VT; *See* Ventricular tachycardia

XYZ leads, 41-42
    for late potential recording, 22-24

Y leads for late potential recording, 22-24

Z leads for late potential recording, 22-24